MW00606354

THE TREATMENT OF DISEASE

BY ACUPUNCTURE

By the same author and publisher

1 SCIENTIFIC ASPECTS OF ACUPUNCTURE
2 ACUPUNCTURE: THE ANCIENT CHINESE ART OF HEALING
3 THE MERIDIANS OF ACUPUNCTURE
4 THE TREATMENT OF DISEASE BY ACUPUNCTURE (this book)
5 ATLAS OF ACUPUNCTURE
6 ACUPUNCTURE: CURE OF MANY DISEASES

Book 1 is written for doctors. It is an attempt to explain acupuncture in terms of science.
Books 2 to 5 explain acupuncture in the traditional Chinese manner and are suitable for doctors and others interested in Far Eastern philosophy and medicine. Book 2 is a general introduction, whilst books 3 to 5 describe specific aspects.
Books 1 to 5 taken together, constitute a Textbook of Acupuncture.
Book 6 is for the non-medical reader, who wants a grasp of the essentials of acupuncture in a few hours.

THE
TREATMENT
OF DISEASE
by

ACUPUNCTURE

Part I FUNCTION OF ACUPUNCTURE POINTS
Part II TREATMENT OF DISEASES

by FELIX MANN

MB, B.chir. (*Cambridge*)
LMCC
Founder of The Medical Acupuncture Society

*Based on the case histories and clinical experience of Dr Felix Mann,
with translations from the Chinese by David Owen, Frank Liu and
Felix Mann*

WILLIAM HEINEMANN MEDICAL BOOKS LTD
LONDON

First published	1963
Second Edition	1967
Reprinted (twice)	1972
Third Edition	1974
Reprinted	1975
Reprinted	1976
Reprinted with additions	1980
Reprinted	1985

ISBN 0 433 20308 0

Printed in Great Britain by

REDWOOD BURN LIMITED

Trowbridge, Wiltshire

AUTHOR'S PREFACE

This book is largely based on Chinese tradition, interlaced with my own experience and that of other European doctors, practising acupuncture.

For the past few years I have done very little else than Chinese acupuncture, both in my own practice and at hospital. The majority of patients whom I (or my European colleagues) have treated, have been patients who already have tried orthodox Western medicine, with little or no success, in their particular disease or symptoms. And since a reasonably high proportion of patients treated, (see statistics in my other book)* are cured or alleviated, I think the subject is worthy of the attention of more doctors, for whom this book is primarily designed.

The wealth of clinical material which I have amassed, by specialising in acupuncture for several years, has largely determined what I have included and what I have excluded from this book.

PART I

This section describes those diseases or symptoms, which may be alleviated or cured, by stimulating a specific acupuncture point.

*Acupuncture. The Ancient Chinese Art of Healing. Heinemann Medical. 1962. Referred to elsewhere only as 'Acupuncture'.

If a doctor has a patient, with say, dyspnoea, and the doctor looks up in this section a point where the word dyspnoea is mentioned, and he stimulates this point with a needle; he will be extremely lucky if the patient is any the better — the patient might even be the worse for it. Of primary importance is an understanding, and an ability to assess and use, the basic principles of diagnosis and therapy in acupuncture, as outlined in 'Acupuncture'. The encyclopaedic data mentioned in this book are only of real value when applied according to the basic principles.

The individual symptoms or diseases mentioned, such as dyspnoea, bronchitis, etc., should not be taken too literally, out of context. The general picture given by the summation of all the individual symptoms or signs of a particular point is of prime importance. It is this general picture, of what a specific acupuncture point is capable of curing or alleviating, that the doctor practicing acupuncture should keep in mind. Obviously it is impossible to remember all the facts mentioned in this section; even if it could be done, it would be of far greater importance to have a vivid, living, general picture of what a specific acupuncture point does — something that can best be gained by long experience coupled with an artistic feeling.

The major part of the description of each point is taken directly from the Chinese books mentioned in the bibliography — mainly the first few. These I read, or at least partly read, while learning to read the largely archaic Chinese that acupuncture books are written in. Not the whole of this section was covered in this way, the remainder being translated by David Owen.

A few of the diseases or symptoms mentioned by the Chinese, cannot in my experience be successfully treated — or at least only rarely. I have therefore reduced, (not omitted, as I may be wrong), the frequency with which these diseases or symptoms are mentioned in my text.

I have tended to oscillate between a literal translation of the Chinese and the nearest Western medical term which is applicable. Often the literal translation of the Chinese is more graphic and hence easier to remember, i.e. 'intestine make sound like thunder', instead of 'borborygmi'; or 'thumping and lurching of the heart' instead of 'palpitations'. Sometimes the Chinese express symptoms in a way, which we by custom do not; 'heart feels hot' or 'Qi (life energy) rushing madly up and down causing pain'; these have often been left literally translated.

In addition to the Chinese description of a point, I have added a few diseases and symptoms, based on my own practical experience.

Before writing down a single disease or symptom I cross-referenced it with at least two other books (entailing a vast amount of work) and added any extra information that thus transpired. Amongst European books I am most indebted to those of A. Chamfrault and S. de Morant, though to a certain extent all European books mentioned in the bibliography of 'Acupuncture', and some of the Chinese mentioned in this book, were used.

The various categories of acupuncture points, to which an individual point belongs, are mentioned under each point, to give a concise description. The terminology used is the same as in 'Acupuncture' except that the Lo points are called Luo after the more modern Chinese system of transliteration. The Gueki (Japanese, in Chinese Hung) have been added, after Y. Manaka. These are points which become tender, on deep pressure, in acute diseases.

The translation of the name of a particular category of point is somewhat arbitrary. I have tended to adhere to the French translation (the Latin root being the same), particularly that of J. E. H. Niboyet, to maintain at least some uniformity. It will be noticed that in a few places the classification clashes. This is unavoidable in a subject that is not completely systematically classified. Some of the categories of points, are in my opinion a natural classification; much as the living world may be classified, with only few exceptions, into the animal and vegetable kingdoms. Other categories, are in my opinion, artificial. I have, however, retained them as a useful aide-mémoire, in the labyrinth of acupuncture.

In common with more recent, standardised, Chinese practice, I have in this book (and in the acupuncture atlas) added one more numbered point between Gv6 and Gv7, the new point being called Gv7; all points above it having their number increased by one, so that the terminal point of the Governing Vessel is Gv28, (instead of Gv27 as in 'Acupuncture'). Also the zig-zag course of the gall bladder meridian on the head has been altered (similarly in the acupuncture charts). This affects several points, though only one, G10 was mentioned in 'Acupuncture'; this becoming G14.

Chinese books, normally give an anatomical description of the position of a point. I have not done this, as I think it is easier to remember a picture than an intricate collection of words. For this reason, I have produced large scale anatomical charts* of acupuncture points, meridians and extra meridians, which I think are more accurate than words can possibly be for this purpose.

PART II

This is the reverse of Part I, being the description of acupuncture points that may be used in a specific disease.

There are of course many more variations than those mentioned, which the experienced acupuncturist tucks away in his subconscious mind, and is able to use when he sees an individual patient, with his individual characteristics, and individual subtle variations. Doctors, who have been to the courses of lecture-demonstrations, which I give to doctors and medical students who wish to study acupuncture, will notice that I have certain preferences and tend to use one technique more than another, as I find that certain techniques give better results.

SECTION 1

This is a translation of Changjian Jibing Zhenjiu Zhiliao Bianlan (A General Survey of Common Diseases and their Treatment by Acupuncture), made by David Owen. To this he has written his own preface overleaf, of the difficulties of translating this subject.

Whilst studying medical Chinese, I read through part of this book, elucidating at the time, most of the practical medical difficulties. This translation was

---

*These have now been replaced by my 'Atlas of Acupuncture'. Heinemann Medical 1966.

good enough for my own purposes, but not precise enough for anyone else to understand. Hence David Owen has retranslated it, trying to make nebulosities that one understands oneself, clear to the reader.

It is divided into five columns:—

Cause of Disease — in the Chinese sense.

Symptoms.

Diagnostic features.

Main Acupuncture Points, that may be used.

Secondary Acupuncture Points, that may be used.

As far as I know, this is the first European book, where the classification and treatment of diseases has really been portrayed following the Chinese system of describing diseases. Other books, have imposed the Western system of medicine on the subject, which, of course, makes it easier and more acceptable to the Western trained doctor, but he has to pay the price of simplification.

If we wish to understand acupuncture fully, we should try and do so in the way that the ancient Chinese did, in their own terminology, trying to think as they thought. Western trained doctors are apt to understand everything in their own terminology — the so-called scientific method — but have a mental blockage when subjects are explained in an entirely different way.

SECTION 2

I have written this section as an addition to Section 1, in an abbreviated style, mentioning only the name of the disease or symptom.

The majority of the points mentioned are ones that I have used in my own practice or at hospital. I have restricted myself as much as I possibly could, to combinations of acupuncture points which I have successfully used.

The more common combinations have been written down from memory, the more rarely used ones, have been looked up in the case history cards of patients whom I have successfully treated for that particular disease or symptom. This does not mean that all these ideas originated in my own mind, though some of them of course did. The others I learnt elsewhere: — from my original teachers, Doctors Johannes Bischko, Anton Strobl and Nguyen Van Nha; from most European authors, particularly the translations from Chinese of A. Chamfrault and G. Soulie de Morant, and of course from Chinese authors direct. All are mentioned in the bibliography of both of my books.

In this section I have classified diseases in a Western way and have put them under the most suitable Chinese heading that I could find, to facilitate reference, even though without the Chinese I would have classified them differently.

Some diseases such as cholera, of which I have no experience, I have not mentioned. A few of which I have little experience have been taken from the sources mentioned above. Some of the children's diseases which may be treated in a similar way (though with a much smaller stimulus), to related adult conditions, have only numbers referring to the adult condition.

LONDON, W.1., 1962   FELIX MANN

INTRODUCTION TO CHINESE TERMINOLOGY

This section has now been transferred to Chapters IV and X of the 2nd (not 1st) edition of Acupuncture: The Ancient Chinese Art of Healing. In that way the subject is more fully integrated with the theoretical framework of traditional acupuncture. It is also described in greater detail.

PREFACE TO SECOND EDITION

In this edition the numbering of the first eight points on the stomach meridian have been altered, to follow more closely the dermatomes of the face. This is consistent with the practice in China.

Many of the 'reunion' points have been changed in accordance with the best Chinese sources. The reunion points in this book and in The Meridians of Acupuncture are now the same.

The translation of some of the names of the acupuncture points has been improved.

Some diseases, signs and symptoms have been added to Part I.

LONDON, W.1., 1967   FELIX MANN

PREFACE TO THIRD EDITION

In this edition two new sections have been added:

The first is a translation of a book by Ye Siu-ting. The original Chinese contains a long description of each disease, similar to that in a textbook of medicine. Western doctors will of course already know all this, or if they have forgotten it may refer to their favourite textbook. For this reason we have only translated the name of the disease and the acupuncture points that may be used in its treatment, though of course the whole Chinese section was originally read. I have found the combinations of acupuncture points mentioned in this book, better than in most, and have therefore added it to my book to make it available to Western readers.

The second new section concerns periosteal acupuncture, which I have evolved over the past years.

LONDON, W.1., 1973   FELIX MANN

It should never be forgotten, that a knowledge of medicine is required to practise acupuncture satisfactorily: it is not the only pre-requisite, but it is an important keystone. A doctor who has studied physiology and pathology, who knows the natural course of a disease, and who has during his studies and practice accumulated a wealth of clinical experience, may tackle a large variety of mild and serious diseases, for he knows what to expect if a given organ is stimulated.

The numerous practitioners of acupuncture, who are not doctors, who do not know the basic principles of medicine, who often have not studied acupuncture adequately, unfortunately, all too often, achieve results commensurate with their lack of knowledge.

PREFACE TO TRANSLATION OF PART II SECTION 1

Chinese is never an easy language to translate, however well one may understand the original. In this case the fact that the bulk of the terminology has remained standardised for anything up to three thousand years, while the language itself has, obviously, developed, means that there may be a considerable difference between what a given word means in modern Chinese and what it means as a technical term in acupuncture, defined as it was, some thousands or hundreds of years ago in the great classics of Chinese medicine from the Nei Jing down. Although an increasing number of modern works on acupuncture are appearing in Chinese, the number of quotations from much earlier works is still considerable, and there is no attempt to revise the terminology or indeed to define it in modern terms. Where definitions exist they are invariably given in archaic terms which are themselves not clear; and they are generally supported by a classical quotation which is by no means always helpful, since the classical language was an extremely terse, epigrammatic and to us who think differently not a clearly defined vehicle of communication.

Another technical difficulty with this particular work is that it is written, as it has been translated, in an abbreviated style, almost in note form. Since Chinese is an almost totally uninflected language, the indications of what part of speech a particular word plays in a given context are fewer here than usual. Normally one relies, as one does very largely in English, but more so, on word order, but in so shortened a style the syntactical structures largely disappear. Most Chinese words are capable of fulfilling more than one grammatical function, and at times it has been a question of choosing a translation which offers the greatest chance of being understood.

By far the greatest obstacle to an acceptable translation, however, has been the relative lack of precedent in English or in other European languages. This is particularly true of the theoretical aspects of the subject, and has meant that generally few accepted equivalents have been available. Words with a capital letter, are mentioned in the Introduction to Chinese Terminology or the Glossary. In some cases it has been found quite impossible to find an English equivalent and the Chinese word has been retained in romanised form, using the Han-yu Pin-yin system.

There are certain unusual phrases which recur throughout the 'symptoms' column. 'Chest melancholy', 'heart troubled', 'abdomen full and melancholy' etc., are common, and I have refrained from writing each with a capital letter since this would leave very few words uncapitalised. The most common however, have been included in the Glossary. In fact these phrases become clearer if one actually is feeling what is described or if that feeling can be remembered. The description of various sensations, which one cannot call 'pain' is by no means easy, and in the West are usually ignored. They are, though, considered of great importance by the Chinese. These descriptions have therefore been translated almost literally, rather than as more generalised terms such as 'lethargy' 'general fatigue' etc. They probably appear all the more strange since the sensation is attributed directly to the particular organ or area of the body; e.g. 'heart melancholy' may be less acceptable than 'a melancholic feeling in the heart' but what the Chinese in fact say is 'heart (is) melancholy'.

SOURCES

Most of what I know of acupuncture I have learned directly from Dr Felix Mann or from his book, 'Acupuncture. The Ancient Chinese Art of Healing'. The Introduction to Chinese Terminology, the Notes to some sections of the translation, and the Glossary, I have taken from:—
Zhongyi Changyong Mingci Jianshi (A brief explanation of common terms in Chinese medicine); compiled by the Academy of Chinese Medicine of Chengdu; published by the Sichuan People's Publishing House, Chengdu 1959. (abbreviated throughout as JIANSHI).

Zhongyixue Gailun (A summary of Chinese medicine); compiled by the Academy of Chinese Medicine of Nanking; published by the People's Hygiene Publishing House, Peking, 1959.

Zhenjiuxue Jiangyi (Lectures in Acupuncture and Moxibustion) compiled by the Acupuncture Research Section of the Shanghai Academy of Chinese Medicine; published by the Shanghai Scientific and Technical Publishing House, Shanghai, 1960.

D. T. OWEN

CONTENTS

PART II. TREATMENT OF DISEASES.

SECTION 1 (CAPITALS) of each disease, is a translation of Changjian Jibing Zhenjiu Zhiliao Bianlan.

SECTION 2 (ordinary print) of each disease, represents acupuncture points taken from the case histories of the author, and other, mainly European, sources.

General Diseases

Diseases of Women

Diseases of Children

PART I

Function of Acupuncture Points

TAKEN FROM ANCIENT AND MODERN SOURCES
(CHINESE AND EUROPEAN), AND THE CASE
HISTORIES OF THE AUTHOR

Lung

Lung 1
ZHONG FU   MIDDLE MANSION

Point of alarm
Point of entry
Meeting point (greater Yin)

Dyspnoea, fullness of chest, oppression, intermittent fever with cough, adenitis, purulent bronchitis, bronchiectasis or pneumonia, pleurisy, pain in chest on respiration, turbid phlegm, anorexia, rheumatism of neck chest and shoulder, tonsillitis, rhinorrhoea, stuttering, oedema of face and limbs, painful skin, acne, sweating at night, insomnia, sensation that energy rises to top of body, eyes red, urine has bad smell.

Lung 2
YUN MEN   CLOUD DOOR

'Harmful cold causing limbs to become hot', bouts of coughing, short of breath, feeling of oppression and pain in chest, asthma, fullness of chest, rheumatism and swelling of neck, tonsillitis, cannot raise arm, neuralgia of shoulder, sensation that energy rises, acne, general cardiac disease.

Lung 3
TIAN FU   HEAVENLY MANSION

Point 'Window of the sky'

Epistaxis, cerebral congestion, speaks to himself or does not speak at all, 'possessed by a devil', confused, forgetful, vertigo, depressed, very thirsty, vomiting, frog in throat, food sticks in throat, dyspnoea, bronchitis, likes to lie down, brachial neuralgia, intermittent fever, carbon monoxide poisoning.

Lung 4
XIA BAI   CHIVALRY WHITE

Rheumatic pains of the chest, cardiac pain, nausea, annoyed, melancholia, skin mottled red and white with excessive perspiration.

Lung 5

CHI ZE FOOT MARSH

Water point
Category VI
Point of sedation

Cold and spasm of arm, bronchitis, pleurisy, cough with turbid mucus, haemoptysis, dyspnoea, sneezing, palpitations, body generally painful, rheumatism of throat and neck, tonsillitis, Wind disease of children, eyes not steady, fever of the five viscera, hemiplegia, quadriplegia, muscular spasm, rigidity of vertebral column, madness, renal pain, atony of the bladder.

Lung 6

KONG ZUI SUPREME HOLE

Accumulation point

High fever with no perspiration, headache, migraine, fear-tension headaches, sore throat, loss of voice, cough, haemoptysis, pain in shoulder and arm.

Lung 7

LIE QUE LISTING DEFICIENCY

Luo point
General Luo point
Point of exit
Master point of Ren mo
Coupled point of Yin qiao
mo

Pain on one side of head or face, trigeminal neuralgia, toothache, migraine, unable to open mouth or speak, tic douloureux, cough with thick mucus, influenza, cough, breathless, melancholic feeling in lower part of chest, trembling, petit mal, epilepsy, mad laughter, yawning, bad memory, middle of palm hot and painful, neuralgia of shoulder and arm with shaking of upper limb, hemiplegia, shivering, cold in the back, limbs ice cold, haematuria, spermatorrhea, pain in penis, haemorrhoids, stye, pruritis, dry skin.

Lung 8

JING QU MERIDIAN GUTTER

Metal point of Yin
metal meridian
Category V

Cough, feeling that energy rises to top of body, intermittent fever, fever without perspiration, sudden onset of cardiac pain, rheumatism of neck, tonsillitis, pharyngitis, spasm of the oesophagus, palm of hand hot.

Lung 9

TAI YUAN BIGGER ABYSS

Earth point
Category III & IV

Conjunctivitis, keratitis, suddenly cold and suddenly hot, feeling that energy rises to top of body, scapula neuralgia, pain in arm and armpit, asthma,

Point of tonification
Source point
Reunion arteries and
veins

dyspnoea, wailing noise with respiration, pain pulmonary and cardiac region, emphysema, haemoptysis, intercostal neuralgia, brachial neuralgia, claustrophobia, facial paralysis, migraine, insomnia, thirsty, dry mouth, nausea, vomiting, faecal incontinence, oesophageal spasm.

Lung 10

YU JI   FISH BORDER

Fire point
Category II

Throat dry and thirsty, cough, muscular spasm of arm, dyspnoea, heart 'numb', mucus streaked with blood, throat hot and swollen, aphonia, aphasia, upset stomach, cholera, yellow tongue, anorexia, aerophagia, headache, vertigo, insomnia, result of alcoholism, breast abscess.

Lung 11

SHAO SHANG   YOUNG MERCHANT

Wood point
Category I
Last point

Throat and jaws swollen, cerebral congestion, meningitis, intermittent fever, tonsillitis, parotitis, epistaxis, hand and arm numb, swollen chest, lips dry, no mucus or saliva, throat and tongue glistening, nocturnal perspiration, shivering, spasms in frightened children, epilepsy.

Large Intestine

Large Intestine 1

SHANG YANG   MERCHANT YANG

*Metal point of Yang
metal meridian
Category I
First point*

'Dyspnoeic feeling in middle of chest', cough, swollen limbs, fever without perspiration, sudden attacks of fever, tinnitus, deafness, mouth dry, jaws swollen, adenitis of face, neck swollen, throat feels as if it is blocked, stomatitis, laryngitis, toothache, membrane over eye, colour blindness, cerebral congestion.

Large Intestine 2

ER JIAN   SECOND INTERVAL

*Water point
Category II
Point of sedation (main)*

Epistaxis, jaundice, toothache, throat numb, tonsillitis, spasm of oesophagus, 'vision confused', inner canthus of eye diseased, headache, renal pain, pain in shoulder and arm, facial palsy, shivering, tongue tired, intestinal colic or spasm, diarrhoea due to inflammatory causes.

Large Intestine 3

SAN JIAN   THIRD INTERVAL

*Wood point
Category III
Point of sedation
(secondary)*

Throat numb, throat blocked, tonsillitis, pain in eye, palpebral pruritis, dyspnoea, brings up much mucus, mouth dry, tongue swollen, lips cracked, diarrhoea, toothache, brachial neuralgia, likes to stretch himself.

Large Intestine 4

HE GU   JOINING OF THE VALLEYS

*Category IV
Source
Point of entry*

Paralysis of limbs, unable to close lips, epistaxis, bleeding from gums, tonsillitis, intermittent fever, sees spots in front of eyes, weak eyesight, headache, migraine, hemiplegia, neuralgia of scapula back and renal area, deafness, tinnitus, aphonia, mute, dyspnoea, insomnia, nervous depression, night sweats, secondary amenorrhoea, pruritis.

Large Intestine 5
YANG XI   YANG STREAM

Fire point
Category V
Bleeding from a scab in the nose, incoherent speech, mad laughter, 'sees the devil', fever without perspiration, nervous palpitations, eye red, inner canthus painful, headache, hemiplegia with anaesthesia, deafness, tinnitus, tonsillitis, neuralgia of the teeth, cough with the expectoration of much mucus, pruritis.

Large Intestine 6
PIAN LI   INCLINED PASSAGE

Luo point
Dimness of vision, fever, madness, mad speech, throat dry and numb, tonsilitis, epistaxis, deafness, tinnitus, neuralgia of the arm, toothache, retention of urine, constipation.

Large Intestine 7
WEN LIU   WARM CURENT

Accumulation point
Fevers, pain in arm, throat numb, toothache, madness, 'sees devils', swollen tongue, glossitis, sticks tongue out, full of air, good at belching, swollen throat, headache, ulcers o. hand and face, stomatitis, parotitis, tonsillitis.

Large Intestine 8
XIA LIAN   LOWER ANGLE

Anorexia, 'abdomen melancholia', indigestion, abdominal pain, abundant stools, lips dry, headache, hemiplegia, body wastes away, emaciated, tuberculosis, mad speech, urine yellow-red, hernia causing vomiting, breast abscess with discharge, dyspnoea.

Large Intestine 9
SHANG LIAN   UPPER ANGLE

Borborygmi, body yellow, gonorrhoea, knee swollen due to wind and wet, hemiplegia, paralysis of the bladder, loss of sensation in limbs, flatulence, dyspnoea, Wind in the brain with headache, cold feeling in the bones and marrow, this point becomes tender after a lot of brain work.

Large Intestine 10
(SHOU) SAN LI (ARM) THREE MILES
Unable to raise arm, muscular spasm, toothache, pruritis, swelling of neck, adenitis, tonsillitis, indigestion, water brash, hemiplegia, cerebral congestion, pain from loin to navel, pleurisy, poor circulation in extremities.

Large Intestine 11
QU CHI CROOKED POND

Earth point
Category VI
Point of tonification
Upper meeting point Ho
of large intestine

Eyes red, pain in front of ear, toothache, neck swollen painful and hot, cannot speak, madness, epilepsy, hemiplegia, erythema, anaemia, brachial neuralgia, intercostal neuralgia, torticollis, cervical adenitis, pleurisy, pruritis, amenorrhoea, atonic constipation, depression, dreams of uncultivated fields.

Large Intestine 12
ZHOU LIAO ELBOW BONE
Elbow joint feels numb, pain in shoulder, unable to raise arm, arm feels wooden and insensitive.

Large Intestine 13
WU LI FIVE MILES
Feeling of melancholy and pain below the heart, brachial neuralgia, four limbs paralysed, cervical adenitis, cannot see clearly, pneumonia, haemoptysis, peritonitis, very sleepy.

Large Intestine 14
BEI NAO OUTER BONE OF ARM

? Point of Yang wei mo

Stiff neck, cervical adenitis, brachial neuralgia, unable to raise arm, headache, fever, shivering.

Large Intestine 15

JIAN YU   SHOULDER BONE (YU)

Independent associated point of shoulder
Point of Yang qiao mo

Brachial neuralgia, hemiplegia, hypertension, muscular spasm in arm and hand, fever of long duration after influenza, spermatorrhoea, dry skin.

Large Intestine 16

JU GU   GREAT BONE

Point of Yang qiao mo

Agitation, epilepsy convulsions in children, brachial neuralgia, haematemesis, toothache.

Large Intestine 17

TIAN DING   HEAVENLY VESSEL

Suddenly dumb, throat numb and painful, tonsillitis, pharyngitis.

Large Intestine 18

FU TU   SUPPORT AND RUSH

Point 'Window of the sky'

Cough, short of breath, stridor, suddenly dumb, hypersalivation, laryngeal spasm, orbital neuralgia, trembling of upper lip, pain in opposite hip.

Large Intestine 19

HE LIAO   GRAIN BONE

Nose obstructed, nasal catarrh, deviation of mouth, muscular spasm of face, epistaxis, catarrhal deafness, nasal polyp, anosmia, parotitis.

Large Intestine 20

YING XIANG   WELCOME FRAGRANCE

Point of exit
Meeting point sunlight Yang

Anosmia, coryza, rhinorrhoea, dry mouth, loss of sensitivity of face, nasal polyp, nose blocked, epistaxis, swollen face, dyspnoea.

Stomach

Stomach 1
CHENG QI   RECEIVE TEARS

Reunion S, Cv
Point of Yang qiao mo
Greenish membrane covers eyes, poor vision, eyes twitch and water, dislikes strong light, cannot see well at night, deafness, tinnitus, facial spasm.

Stomach 2
SI BAI   FOUR WHITES

Headache, eyes feel dizzy, membrane over eye, eyes blink, eyes water easily, orbital neuralgia, eyes feel as if they have smoke in them, allergic rhinorrhoea, facial spasm, cannot speak.

Stomach 3
JU LIAO   GREAT BONE

Reunion S, Li
Point of Yang qiao mo
Nose blocked due to wind and cold, rhinorrhoea, abscess of the nose, maxillary sinusitis, weak distant vision, nystagmus, blepharospasm, convulsions, facial paralysis, dental neuralgia, aphonia, swelling of the jaw and lips, swelling and rheumatism of the feet.

Stomach 4
DI CANG   EARTH GRANARY

Reunion S, Li
Point of Yang qiao mo
Suddenly dumb, cannot speak, laryngitis, general catarrhal condition, neuralgia and paralysis of the face, cannot close his eyelids or blink, cannot see clearly at night, nystagmus, swelling of the feet.

Stomach 5
DA YING   BIG WELCOME

Reunion S, G
Neck painful, glandular swelling, stiffness of the tongue, cannot speak, mad

fits, fits due to Wind, dry mouth, nystagmus, eyes blink, facial spasm, neuralgia of teeth in lower jaw, parotitis, fever with shivering.

Stomach 6

JIA CHE   JAW CHARIOT

Reunion S, G Jaw swollen, cannot speak, laryngitis, dental neuralgia, glaucoma, myopia, sees spots in front of eyes, neck rigid, difficult to turn, spasm of facial muscles, trigeminal neuralgia, acne of face.

Stomach 7

XIA GUAN   LOWER GATE

? Reunion S, G Tinnitus, deafness, otitis externa, orbital neuralgia, feels as if smoke in eyes, poor distant vision, eyes red and painful, foggy distant vision, headache, vertigo, yawning, fainting, facial neuralgia or spasm, maxilla that easily dislocates, pyorrhea, teeth that are loose.

Stomach 8

TOU WEI   HEAD TIED

Point of entry Headache, head feels as if it is broken, facial paralysis, hemiplegia, loss of sensa-
? Reunion S, G tion in face, dyspnoea, pain in eye, eye feels as if it has been pulled out, eyes water, dislikes sunlight, conjunctivitis, blinking of eyelids, pain above eyelids.

Stomach 9

REN YING   MAN WELCOME

Point 'Window of the Fullness of the chest, dyspnoea, throat swollen red and painful, cervical
sky' adenitis, pharyngitis, tonsillitis, vomiting, feeling as if energy under high
Sea of energy tension shoots up and down.

Stomach 10

SHUI TU   WATER RUSHING

Dyspnoea, Qi in upper part of body, tonsillitis, pharyngitis, bronchitis, whooping cough, spasmodic cough, pruritis, urticaria.

Stomach 11
QI SHE   QI SHELTER

Throat numb and swollen, neck rigid and painful, dyspnoea, pharyngitis, goitre, swelling of glands in neck, 'energy high'.

Stomach 12
QUE PEN   BROKEN BOWL

Reunion S, Li, T, G, Si   Pain in clavicular fossa, throat numb, cervical adenitis, haemoptysis, incessant cough, middle of chest hot and swollen, dyspnoea, pleurisy, intercostal neuralgia, generalised subcutaneous oedema, excessive loquacity, insomnia due to nervousness.

Stomach 13
QI HU   QI COTTAGE

Chest ribs and limbs heavy, dyspnoea, 'energy high', pleurisy, bronchitis, frequent coughing, spasm of diaphragm, loss of taste and smell, loss of appetite, feet perspire too much.

Stomach 14
KU FANG   STOREHOUSE

Chest ribs and limbs heavy, dyspnoea, 'energy high', sputum thick and streaked with blood, pulmonary congestion, bronchitis, pleurisy, physical and mental consequences of a shock.

Stomach 15
WU YI   ROOM SCREEN

Chest ribs and limbs heavy, little children dyspneic with a swollen belly, whole body itches, dyspneic, asthma, 'energy high', thick phlegm streaked with blood, intercostal neuralgia, melancholic, tumour of the breast.

Stomach 16
YING CHUANG   BREAST WINDOW

Ulcers of the breast, breasts too big, 'chest melancholia', short of breath, emphysema, intercostal neuralgia, fever with sensation of cold, insomnia, swelling of the lips, diarrhoea, bitter taste in mouth, heart-burn.

Stomach 17
RU ZHONG MIDDLE OF BREAST
Most Chinese authors say that this point should not be used. One Chinese author writes that it is recorded in ancient texts that this point cures (or causes?) violent madness.

Chamfrault uses it in all diseases of the nipple.

Stomach 18
RU GEN BREAST ROOT
Chest pain, hiccough, hacking cough, coughing and panting with much phlegm, breast exhausted, not enough milk, retained placenta, menstruation lasting more than nine days.

Stomach 19
BU RONG NO ADMITTANCE
Pain in chest, abdomen melancholic and empty with borborygmi, cough, mouth dry, indigestion with much phlegm and painful ribs, eye diseases of little children, cardiac pain.

Stomach 20
CHENG MAN RECEIVING FULLNESS
Intestinal noises with diarrhoea, lower ribs in the position of full inspiration, dyspnoea, cannot swallow food or drink, jaundice, haemoptysis.

Stomach 21
LIANG MEN BEAM DOOR
Diarrhoea due to colonic disease, cannot use food or drink, anorexia, acute gastritis, all gastric troubles due to excesses, irritable stomach.

Stomach 22
GUAN MEN   GATE DOOR
Abdomen swollen, aerogastria, gastritis, anorexia, intestinal noises and diarrhoea, feverish, shakes with cold, urinary incontinence, oedema, bad breath.

Stomach 23
TAI YI   BIGGER YI (A CELESTIAL STEM)
Mad, walks about madly, neurasthenia, palpitations, sticks out tongue, bad digestion, cold limbs.

Stomach 24
HUA ROU MEN   SLIPPERY MEAT DOOR
Madness, vomiting, haematemesis, tongue rigid, sticks tongue out, glossitis, pain under tongue, dysmenorrhoea.

Stomach 25
TIAN SHU   HEAVENLY PIVOT

Alarm point of large intestine
Shokanten of lesser Yang
Reunion S, Li

Pain round the umbilicus, abdomen bloated, borborygmi, weary, frightened, weak, bowel disease in men, aqueous stools, irregular menstruation, leucorrhoea, sterility in women, dysentery with stabbing pain, retention of urine, ? oedema, ascites — the last two conditions are not altered by food or drink.

Stomach 26
WAI LING   OUTSIDE MOUND
Lower end of heart feels as if it is suspended, pain around umbilicus, intestinal spasm, spasm of rectus abdominus.

Stomach 27
DA JU   BIG GREAT

Shokanten of Sunlight Yang

Hernia, lower abdomen swollen and full, premature ejaculation, insomnia, weakness of limbs, constipation.

Stomach 28
SHUI DAO   WATER PATH
Triple warmer hot and congealed (genito-urinary function of lower triple warmer), retention of urine and faeces, lower abdomen distended, nephritis, cystitis, rectal prolapse, uterine and ovarian disease, inflamation of scrotum, pain going into vagina.

Stomach 29
GUI LAI   THE RETURN
'Hurrying and shuffling' in the lower abdomen, shrunken scrotum, pain in penis, orchitis, uterus cold, amenorrhoea, leucorrhoea, sterility. This point has a special effect on the male and female genitalia.

Stomach 30
QI CHONG   RUSHING QI

Centre reunion particular point of food
Sea of nourishment
Reunion S, G
Point of Chong mo

Abdominal pain, spasm in foot, unable to use foot, hernia, swelling of penis, pain in penis, impotent, 'uterine cloths' (placenta) retained, amenorrhoea, menorrhagia, energy that rises to top of body, sensation of warmth in stomach.

Stomach 31
BI GUAN   THIGH GATE
Pain in loins and knee, lower limbs feel numb — like wood, paralysis of limbs, muscular cramp, inguinal adenitis, gonorrhoea, pain in the lower abdomen radiating to the throat.

Stomach 32
FU TU   PROSTRATE HARE

Reunion of veins

Loins thighs and legs painful, knee cold not warm, atrophy of arm, uterine trouble, head heavy, abdomen distended, very mild varicose veins, oedema of legs, asthma in the middle of the night.

Stomach 33
YIN SHI   YIN MARKET
Painful hernia, pain in abdomen, paralysis and numbness of limbs, spasm and cramp in feet, ascites, very thirsty, uterine spasm, irregular menstruation, trembling hands, no energy.

Stomach 34
Accumulation point

LIANG QIU   BEAM MOUND
Pain in loins knees and feet, limbs cold and numb, stomach pain and cramp, breast swollen and painful.

Stomach 35
DU BI   CALF NOSE
Pain in knee, unable to bend knee, rheumatism of feet, oedema of feet due to humidity.

Stomach 36
(ZU) SAN LI   (LEG) THREE MILES

Earth point of Yang earth meridian Category VI Centre reunion particular point of energy Lower meeting point Ho of stomach Sea of nourishment Reunion of energy

Globus hystericus, gastritis, anorexia, intestinal noises, abdominal pain, abdomen swollen, anuria, food does not change abdominal pain, indigestion, constipation, appendicitis — slightly below S36, weak limbs, agitated and emaciated, general lack of energy, tinnitus, eye diseases, nervousness, difficulty in speaking.

Some books mention practically every disease under this point.

Stomach 37
SHANG JU XU   UPPER GREAT VOID

Lower meeting point

Chest ribs and limbs swollen, arthritis of knee, intestinal noises, diarrhoea,

Ho of large intestine
Sea of blood

hemiplegia, unable to raise hand or foot, spleen and stomach empty and weak, gastritis, colitis, anorexia, marrow of the bone feels cold.

Stomach 38
TIAO KOU LINE MOUTH
Weakness of legs, hemiplegia, loss of sensation in limbs and renal area, rheumatism caused by humidity, tonsillitis, gastritis, entero-colitis, diarrhoea.

Stomach 39
XIA JU XU LOWER GREAT VOID

Lower meeting point Ho
of the small intestine
Sea of blood

Pain in lower abdomen associated with diarrhoea, pain in loins and legs, diseases of the breast, madness, cerebral anaemia, generalised aches and pains in body, intercostal neuralgia, tonsillitis, hypersalivation, lips dry, no sweat, loss of hair.

Stomach 40
FENG LONG ABUNDANT BULGE

Luo point

Throat numb, cannot speak, headache, swollen face, dyspnoea with much phlegm and coughing, asthma hindering sleep, paralysis of leg, constipation, oliguria, madness, sees ghosts, laughs madly.

Stomach 41
JIE XI DISSOLVE STREAM

Fire point
Category V
Point of tonification

Head and face swollen, toothache, gingivitis, vertigo, madness, fits, convulsions in children, stomach hot with incoherent speech, eyes red with headache, muscles numb, rheumatism of feet, frightened and agitated.

Stomach 42
CHONG YANG RUSHING YANG

Category IV
Source

Fever without perspiration, always cold, seeks warmth, wants to undress in public, walks around aimlessly, 'every month madness', wishes to climb on to tables etc. and sing, paralysis of foot, toothache, gingivitis, anorexia, vomiting, yawning.

Stomach 43

XIAN GU SINKING VALLEY

Wood point
Category III
Chest ribs and limbs heavy, face swollen, congestion of eyes, thirsty with indigestion and fever, ascites, abdomen swollen with much belching, coughing that does not stop, very high fever.

Stomach 44

NEI TING INNER COURT YARD

Water point
Category II
Pain around navel, abdomen distended, asthmatic and melancholic, pain with fear and trembling, nightmares, dislikes the human voice, toothache, gingivitis, epistaxis, throat numb, anorexia, diarrhoea — the motion having pus and blood, skin rash and pustules with intermittent fever, dysmenorrhoea.

Stomach 45

LI DUI GENERAL EXCHANGE

Metal point
Category I
Point of sedation
Last point
Fainting, cerebral anaemia, 'like a corpse', deviation of mouth, face swollen, epistaxis, acute rhinitis, cold nose, sinusitis, throat numb, tonsillitis, fever with no perspiration, toothache, epigastrium swollen, eyes twitch, madness awaking and sleeping all the time with many dreams.

Spleen

Spleen 1
YIN BAI   HIDDEN WHITE

Wood point
Category I
Point of entry

Dyspnoea, asthma, abdomen swollen, little children cantankerous, severe vomiting, thirsty, hyperacidity, menorrhagia, epistaxis, haemorrhoids, foot cold and paralysed, madness, cannot remain still in bed.

Spleen 2
DA DU   BIG CAPITAL

Fire point
Category II
Point of tonification

'Humors of the body hot', spermatorrhoea, abdomen distended, agitated, melancholic, indigestion, does not absorb food, epigastric pain, spasm of stomach, general fatigue, body heavy, lumbago, limbs cold, cannot remain still in bed, foggy vision.

Spleen 3
TAI BAI   SUPREME WHITENESS

Earth point of Yin earth
meridian
Category III & IV
Source

Fever, melancholic, agitated, chest ribs and abdomen swollen, intestinal noises with stabbing pain, diarrhoea, intestinal haemorrhage, constipation, diarrhoea with pus and blood, mad, body heavy, lumbago, haemorrhoids cardiac pain, cold feet.

Spleen 4
GONG SUN   GRANDFATHER GRANDSON

Luo point
Master point of Chong
mo
Coupled point of Yin wei
mo

Intestine swollen, stabbing pain in intestines, abdomen swollen, ascites, cardiac pain, pleurisy, vomits foul food, intestinal haemorrhage, fever with yellow ulcers and excessive perspiration, face swollen, very thirsty.

Spleen 5

SHANG QIU   MERCHANT MOUND

Metal point
Category V
Point of sedation
Reunion of veins

Vomits a lot, a gourmand — but cannot digest his food, headache, swollen face, spleen empty, indigestion, pain along inside of thighs, hernia, abdominal pain, agitation in little children, dreams of ghosts, sighs often, haemorrhoids, spasm in feet, yellow ulcer, yellow urine, jaundice, sterility.

Spleen 6

SAN YIN JIAO   THREE YIN CROSSING

Group Luo point of 3
lower Yin
Reunion Sp, K, Liv

All diseases of the genitalia of both sexes, menorrhagia, spermatorrhoea, pain in genitalia, abdomen swollen, diarrhoea, symptoms not changed by food or drink, chest in position of inspiration with phlegm and cough, dysuria, retained foetus, foot paralysed numb or painful, haemorrhoids, insomnia, nervous depression.

Spleen 7

LOU GU   LEAKY VALLEY

Abdomen swollen, borborygmi, indigestion, flatulence, eats much without gaining weight, numbness, not able to walk, very little urine, mad, foot and ankle swollen and painful.

Spleen 8

DI JI   EARTH ORGAN

Accumulation point

Abdomen swollen, ascitis, anorexia, spermatorrhoea, irregular menstruation, leucorrhoea, very little urine, haemorrhoids, lumbago, intermittent fever.

Spleen 9

YIN LING QUAN   YIN MOUND SPRING

Water point
Category VI

Water swelling eliminates umbilicus — ascites, spermatorrhoea, very little urine, pain in loins and knees, chest ribs and abdomen heavy, intermittent fever, dyspnoea, dysmenorrhoea, weakness of legs, cramps.

Spleen 10
XUE HAI   SEA OF BLOOD
Dysmenorrhoea, menorrhagia, metritis, oligomenorrhoea, orchitis, perineal eczema, indigestion.

Spleen 11
JI MEN   BASKET DOOR
Very little urine, incontinence of urine, gonorrhoea, inguinal adenitis.

Spleen 12
CHONG MEN   RUSHING DOOR

Reunion Sp, Liv   Abdomen swollen and painful, gastric spasm, retention of urine, hernia, haemorrhoids, dyspnoea, menorrhagia, dysmenorrhoea, orchitis, epididy-mitis, insufficient milk, breast abscess, rectal prolapse.

Spleen 13
FU SHE   MANSION COTTAGE

Reunion Sp, Liv   Hernia, pain in buttocks, indigestion, intestinal spasm, abdominal pain.
Point of Yin wei mo

Spleen 14
FU JIE   ABDOMEN KNOT
Periumbilical pain, abdominal pain, diarrhoea, heart agitated, cough, dyspnoea, weakness of legs, excessive perspiration.

Spleen 15
DA HENG   BIG HORIZONTAL

Point of Yin wei mo   Unable to use limbs, excessive perspiration, influenza, constipated, entero-colitis, always sad.

Spleen 16
FU AI   ABDOMEN SORROW

Point of Yin wei mo Intestinal haemorrhage, blood in stools, pus in stools, periumbilical pain, symptoms not altered by food or drink, peptic ulcer, hypo or hyperacidity.

Spleen 17
SHI DOU   FOOD DRAIN

Chest ribs and limbs heavy, diaphragmatic pain, intestines make sound like thunder, intermittent fever of the spleen, paralysis and numbness, ascites, pulmonary congestion.

Spleen 18
TIAN XI   HEAVENLY STREAM

Middle of chest full and painful, bronchitis, breast swollen and large, insufficient milk, rebellious cough, throat noises, peptic ulcer.

Spleen 19
XIONG XIANG   CHEST VILLAGE

Chest ribs and limbs heavy, bronchitis, loss of appetite, difficulty in lying down or turning.

Spleen 20
ZHOU RONG   ENCIRCLING GLORY

Chest ribs and abdomen distended, cough, 'energy high', purulent and blood stained sputum, haemorrhoids, eyelids swollen.

Spleen 21
DA BAO   BIG ENVELOPING

Luo point of all Luo points
Point of exit Dyspnoea with chest pain, pain on one side of head and body while other side is relaxed; harmonises right and left, upper and lower, inside and outside of body.

Heart

Heart 1
JI QUAN   EXTREME SPRING

Point of Entry   Inflammation of the heart, dry throat, cardiac pain, very thirsty, pain in the chest and ribs, feeling of fullness in chest, spasm of the chest, 'frog in throat', nausea, hysteria, moral depression, hypotension, paralysis of all limbs, forearm cold, tip of tongue tender or numb, eyesight weak, excessive perspiration due to weakness, too impulsive.

Heart 2
QING LING   GREEN SPIRIT

Dislike of cold, shivering, fever, frontal headache, generalised headache, neuralgia and spasm of arm, unable to raise arm or shoulder, cannot wear clothes, intercostal neuralgia, congestion and feeling of constriction in middle and lower thorax.

Heart 3
SHAO HAI   LESSER SEA

Water point
Category VI   Glandular disease, scrofulous swellings, adenitis, hand and fingers cold, epilepsy, madness, eyes dizzy, diplopia, fainting, bleats like a sheep, toothache, headache due to wind or cold, dizzy, intercostal neuralgia, facial neuralgia, spasm of shoulder or arm, trembling and shaking of hand, pleurisy, torticollis, spasm of elbow, fever with sensation of cold, feels as if energy goes to top part of body, stupidity, forgetfulness, mental depression, coughing up mucus, cannot move limbs, mammary pain, pruritis, trembling in infants, adds stability to nervous exhaustion.

Heart 4

LING DAO SPIRIT PATH

Metal point
Category V
Arthritis of elbow and wrist, spasm and neuralgia of arm, loss of sensation in upper arm, convulsions, hysteria, cardiac pain, fear, anxiety, suddenly mute, unable to speak, paralysis of tongue muscles, nausea, ice cold feeling in bone.

Heart 5

TONG LI PENETRATING INSIDE

Luo point
Headache, eyes dizzy, dizziness, vertigo, palpitations, tonsillitis, sudden dumbness, throat spasm, pharyngitis, neuralgia and spasm of upper limbs and shoulder blade area, hysteria, not happy, anxiety, fear, fear of people, words fall over one another, dysmenorrhoea, metrorrhagia, incontinence of urine, urinary frequency, clear urine, lack of energy, face warm without sweat, yawning, vomiting, conjunctivitis, abdomen swollen, constipation.

Heart 6

YIN HUNG YIN ACCUMULATION

Accumulation point
Epistaxis, nose blocked, dizziness, headache, palpitations, tonsillitis, brachial neuralgia, hysteria, startled, frightened, short of breath, pain in chest, fullness of chest, shivering, leucorrhoea, endometritis, night sweats, haematemesis, fainting, suddenly dumb, tongue without strength, sudden diarrhoea, cannot bend elbow.

Heart 7

SHEN MEN SPIRIT DOOR

Earth point
Category III & IV
Point of sedation
Source
Psychological and physical cardiac diseases, heart big and dilated, warmth and pain in cardiac area, shortness of breath, palpitations, inflammation of the nose, nose blocked, red face, desire for cool drinks, loss of speech, hysteria, shortness of breath with a hot body, face purple and raving, likes to laugh, frightened, laughing and sobbing alternating, hallucinations, loss of taste and appetite, dry throat, tonsillitis, insomnia due to excitement, post-partum

haemorrhage, urinary incontinence, cold feet, fear of cold, shivering, palms of hands warm, cardiac and renal energy weak, sighing, forgetfulness, irregular cardiac rhythm, fibrillation, oedematous tongue, cannot stop talking, cardiac oedema, retention of fluid, cold sweat, migraine.

Heart 8

SHAO FU   LESSER MANSION

Fire point of Yin,
Princely, fire meridian
Category II

Diseases and a feeling of calamity in the heart and chest, palpitations, precordial pain, hysteria, fear, frightened of people, trembling, throat dry, sighing, shivering, intermittent fever, neuralgia and numbness of arm and shoulder, hand contracted — cannot be extended, pain and muscular spasm on front of shoulder and armpit, palm of hand warm, difficulty in urination, urinary incontinence, one side of scrotum larger than the other, impotent, general uterine disease, pruritis vulvae, prolapse of the uterus, metrorrhagia.

Heart 9

SHAO CHONG   LESSER RUSHING

Wood point
Category 1
Point of tonification
Point of exit

General cardiac disease, palpitations, heart weak, atonic, steady pulse, mental discouragement, eyes not clear, expressionless voice, neuralgia of arm from palm to armpit, intercostal neuralgia, pleurisy, fullness of chest, bronchial hypersecretion, pharyngitis, dry throat, fever, weakness after fever, fever with sensation of cold, feeling of energy in upper part of body, vaginal odour, white or red vaginal discharge, dreams of fire and smoke.

Small Intestine

Small Intestine 1
SHAO ZE LESSER MARSH

Metal Point
Category I
Point of Entry

Headache, pharyngitis, cough, tonsillitis, cardiac pain, breathless on exertion, brachial neuralgia, torticollis, pain in chest, agalactia, membrane over eye, diarrhoea, dry mouth, polyuria, epistaxis, convulsions in children.

Small Intestine 2
QIAN GU FRONT VALLEY

Water point
Category II

Intermittent fever, fever without sweating, cough, haematemesis, tonsillitis, throat and cheeks red and swollen, nose blocked, coryza, agalactia, mastitis, brachial neuralgia, not able to lift arm, epilepsy, tinnitus, weak eye sight.

Small Intestine 3
HOU XI BACK STREAM

Wood point
Category III
Point of tonification
Master point of Du mo
Coupled point of Yang qiao mo

Madness, epilepsy, epistaxis, deafness, eye red and painful, white membrane over eye, tonsillitis, spasm and pain in arm and forearm, stiff neck, torticollis, pruritis, night sweats, recovers slowly after a shock, bad digestion, greasy stools.

Small Intestine 4
WAN GU WRIST BONE

Category IV

Arthritis of arm forearm and fingers, pain and spasm of fingers, not able to

Source point bend or stretch fingers, creaking of neck, pharyngitis, white membrane over eye with tears, tinnitus, headache, vomiting, irritated stomach, pleurisy, hemiplegia, convulsions, meningism, apprehension, sense of touch dulled, excessive perspiration, alternately hot and cold.

Small Intestine 5

YANG GU   YANG VALLEY

Fire point of Yang, Dizziness, fainting, tinnitus, deafness, stomatitis, gingivitis, neuralgia of arm
Princely, fire meridian and wrist, cannot raise arm, intercostal neuralgia, weakness, fears and spasm
Category V of children, epilepsy, stiff tongue, children cannot suckle, talks or laughs excessively, painful haemorrhoids.

Small Intestine 6

YANG LAO   SUPPORTING THE OLD

Accumulation point Paralysis and neuralgia of the arm, arm feels as if it is broken and uprooted, unable to raise or lower arm, eyes bloodshot, diminished strength of vision.

Small Intestine 7

ZHI ZHENG   BRANCH STRAIGHT

Luo point Forearm and front of shoulder-spasm and not able to bend or stretch, pain in hand, cannot hold objects, face red and feels dizzy, vertigo, throat swollen, headache, intermittent fever, psychopathic apprehension, fear, cyst of eyelids.

Small Intestine 8

XIAO HAI   SMALL SEA

Earth point Spasm and neuralgia of the whole upper limb, eyes bloodshot, dizzy Wind?
Category VI listening and feeling dulled, gingivitis, dancing madly, tics, trembling,
Point of sedation insanity, cervical adenitis, lower abdominal pain, pulmonary oedema, swell-
Upper meeting point Ho ings, pruritis, shivering.
of small intestine

Small Intestine 9

JIAN ZHEN   SHOULDER CHASTITY

Tinnitus, deafness, headache, neuritis, arthritis and pain of upper limbs and scapula, numbness due to wind, unable to raise hand or foot, fever after having been exposed to wind.

Small Intestine 10

NAO YU   SHOULDER BLADE YU

Independent associated point of shoulder blade Point of Yang wei mo and Yang qiao mo

Shoulder and scapula region: muscular pain, numbness, arthritis, weakness, hot-cold feeling, swelling, unable to raise arm.

Small Intestine 11

TIAN ZONG   HEAVENLY ANCESTOR

Scapula region-neuralgia and numbness, neuralgia of forearm, cannot lift arms, swelling of lower jaw.

Small Intestine 12

BING FENG   FACING THE WIND

Reunion Si, Li, T, G

Shoulder and arm neuralgia and numbness, cannot raise arm, pneumonia, pleurisy.

Small Intestine 13

QU YUAN   CROOKED WALL

Neuralgia and numbness of the shoulder and arm, shoulder hot, unable to embrace.

Small Intestine 14

JIAN WAI YU   OUTSIDE OF THE SHOULDER YU

Independent associated point of the outside of the shoulder

Spasm, muscular pain and neuralgia of shoulder and arm, sensation of coldness encircling shoulder and going as far as elbow, spasm of neck muscles, pneumonia, pleurisy.

Small Intestine 15
JIAN ZHONG YU   MIDDLE OF THE SHOULDER YU
Bronchitis, shortness of breath, mucus streaked with blood, torticollis, weak eye sight.

Small Intestine 16
TIAN CHANG   HEAVENLY WINDOW

Point 'Window of the sky' Half of the body not co-ordinated, aphonia, movements slow and lethargic, not fully under voluntary control, neck slanting to one side, spasm of neck and shoulder, unable to twist neck, intercostal neuralgia, inflammation of jaw, deafness, tinnitus, anal fistula.

Small Intestine 17
TIAN RONG   HEAVENLY APPEARANCE

Point 'Window of the sky' Pleurisy, dyspnoea, sternal pain, intercostal neuralgia, difficulty in straightening body, neuralgia, swelling and immobility of neck, tinnitus, deafness, swollen tongue, gingivitis, nausea, vomiting.

Small Intestine 18
QUAN LIAO   CHEEK BONE

Reunion Si, T, G Trigeminal neuralgia face red, not able to eat, facial neuralgia and numbness, mouth twisted, eyes blinking, eyes that always move, pharyngitis, toothache.

Small Intestine 19
TING GONG   LISTENING PALACE

Point of exit
Reunion Si, T, G Tinnitus, deafness, otitis externa, hoarseness.

Bladder

Bladder 1

JING MING   EYES BRIGHT

Point of entry
Meeting point greater
Yang
Reunion B, S, Si, T, G
Point of Yang and Yin
qiao mo

Eye disease, eyes dizzy, inner canthus red and painful, white membrane over eye, conjunctivitis, tears flow in wind, master point for the eyes, dim vision, retinitis, poor night vision, vertigo, headache.

Bladder 2

ZAN ZHU   DRILLING BAMBOO

Brain tired, stiff neck, madness, eyes red, eyes red and painful with headache, eye lazy, eye wanders, excessive blinking, vision foggy, eyes water, convergent strabismus, hay fever, allergic rhinorrhoea, sneezing especially in light and wind, sinusitis, supraorbital neuralgia, nausea, vomiting, nightmares, hallucination, perspiration acid and rancid.

Bladder 3

MEI CHONG   EYEBROW RUSHING

Headache, fainting, epilepsy, nose blocked, catarrh, not able to smell foul smells, maxillary sinusitis.

Bladder 4

QU CHAI   CROOKED SERVANT

Headache, pain on summit of head, facial neuralgia, burning heat in head, stiff neck, rhinophyma, nose blocked, epistaxis, ulcer in nose, nasal polyp, acute dyspnoea, dislikes sunlight in eyes, weak eyesight, no perspiration.

Bladder 5
WU CHU   FIVE PLACES
Spine rigid, spine arched backwards, headache, eyes dizzy, eyes weak, madness, epilepsy, loss of consciousness, does not recognise people, pain in renal area, pain in cervical and upper thoracic vertebrae, neuralgia of canine teeth, heartburn.

Bladder 6
CHENG GUANG   RECEIVE LIGHT
Fever without perspiration, vomiting, vertigo after a shock, palpitations, white membrane covers eye, keratitis, dim vision, foggy vision, cataract, nose blocked, allergic rhinorrhoea, anosmia, cardiac disease, pain over deltoid.

Bladder 7
TONG TIAN   PENETRATE HEAVEN
Headache, head heavy, torticollis, cervical adenitis, nose blocked, epistaxis, rhinitis, anosmia, face swollen, facial neuralgia, dyspnoea, chronic bronchitis, dry mouth, thirsty, convulsions, vertigo, eyesight weak.

Bladder 8
LUO QUE   CONNECTING DEFICIENT
Epilepsy, falls down and lies as stiff as a corpse, obsessions, walks around madly, head revolves, tinnitus, eyes see dimly, abdomen swollen, rheumatism of neck and shoulder.

Bladder 9
YU ZHEN   JADE PILLOW
Pain in eye and supraorbital region, eyes feel as if they have been torn out, shooting pain in eye on bending or raising head, eyes water in cold wind, dim vision, myopia, vertigo, head and neck heavy and painful, occipital neuralgia, nose blocked, anosmia, grieved, weary, neuralgias, hypertensive encephalopathy.

Bladder 10

TIAN ZHU   HEAVENLY PILLAR

Point 'Window of the sky'
Sea of energy
Supposedly vago-sympathetic

Head heavy, spasm of neck muscles, brachial neuralgia, torticollis, writers cramp, light-headedness, limbs and body not co-ordinated, legs collapse under body, throat swollen, difficulty in speaking, nose blocked, weak sense of smell, epistaxis, neurasthenia, nymphomania, seems to have a regularising effect on medullary functions.

Bladder 11

DA ZHU   BIG SHUTTLE

Sea of blood
Special point for bone
Reunion B, ? Si, ? T, G

High fever without perspiration, influenza, generalised spasms in the body, generalised muscular rheumatism, headache, vertigo, epilepsy, fainting, nervous agitation, chest full, bronchitis, pain in loins, muscular spasm in back, abdominal distension, arthritis of knee, an important point for all osseous diseases, stiffness of the vertebral column.

Bladder 12

FENG MEN   WIND GATE

Reunion B, Gv

Severe muscular spasm of the neck, headache, head feels dizzy, spermatorrhoea, dyspnoeic, cough, asthma, unable to lie down, vomiting, preventative for the after effects of a chill, influenza, fever, tosses about in his bed, delirious with fever, allergic rhinorrhoea, sneezing, epistaxis, acne of the shoulders and back, abscess of the back.

Bladder 13

FEI YU   LUNG YU

Associated point of lung

Cough, asthma, dyspnoea, chest feels heavy, pneumonia, bronchitis, agitated, perspiration, pruritis, vomits, haemoptysis, gastritis, water brash, anorexia, mouth and tongue dry, carditis, bored.

Bladder 14

JUE YIN YU   ABSOLUTE YIN YU

Associated point of circulation — sex

Pleurisy, middle of chest feels agitated and depressed, bouts of coughing, cardiac pain, enlarged heart, vomiting, neuralgia of the teeth especially molars, epistaxis, sunstroke, heatstroke, mountain sickness.

Bladder 15

XIN YU   HEART YU

Associated point of heart

Palpitations with shortness of breath, cannot sleep lying down, cardiac pain, easily sad, haemoptysis, vomiting, madness, eyesight poor, body empty and weak, face as red as a beetroot, body below heart feels dead, impotence, perspiration localised over sternum, cannot stop talking, wishes of heart and brain not co-ordinated.

Bladder 16

DU YU   GOVERNING VESSEL YU

Associated point of governing vessel

Cardiac pain, dilatation of heart, hiccough, flatulence, colic, borborygmi, abdominal pain, pain in loins, fever with shivering, nervous breakdown.

Bladder 17

GE YU   DIAPHRAGM YU

Associated point of diaphragm
Centre reunion general point of Yang and Yin and blood

Cardiac pain, throat numb, carditis, body feels empty weary and emaciated, vomiting of food, does not digest food, haemoptysis, gastritis, anorexia, enteritis, chest and abdomen distend 'hot blooded,', night sweats, pleurisy, dyspnoea.

Bladder 18

GAN YU   LIVER YU

Associated point of liver

Haemoptysis, dyspnoea, chest and ribs full and melancholic, enlarged liver, dark rings round eyes, epistaxis, pale stools, bitter taste in mouth, jaundice, duodenal ulcer, bad tempered, haemorrhoids, angio-neurotic oedema, intercostal neuralgia, bronchitis, asthma.

Bladder 19

DAN YU   GALL BLADDER YU

Associated point of gall bladder

Weary, fever, shivering, choleric, dry mouth, bitter taste in mouth, jaundice, pain in lower ribs, epigastrium distended, haemoptysis, vomits food, hypertension, pleurisy, eyebrows tender, eyes yellow, eyes bloodshot.

Bladder 20

PI YU   SPLEEN YU

Associated point of spleen

Chest painful, abdomen protruding, oesophogeal and tracheal pain, colitis, gastritis, indigestion, vomits dark food, eats a lot but remains thin, poor digestion, anorexia, diarrhoea, undigested stools, defective night vision, intermittent fever.

Bladder 21

WEI YU   STOMACH YU

Associated point of the stomach

Stomach ache, borborygmi, gastric haemorrhage, vomiting, diarrhoea, stool mixed with pus and blood, abdomen swollen, gastritis, flatulence, green stools in children, regurgitation of milk, eats a lot but remains thin, anorexia, poor eyesight, does not see well at dusk, dyspnoea, limbs heavy.

Bladder 22

SAN JIAO YU   TRIPLE WARMER YU

Associated point of triple warmer

Bowels 'congealed', borborygmi, distended abdomen, enterocolitis, anorexia, melaena, flatulence, cannot digest food, pain in loins, incontinence of urine, feeling of tightening in back and shoulder, stiff vertebral column.

Bladder 23

SHEN YU   KIDNEY YU

Associated point of kidney

Weary, empty, emaciated, deafness due to the kidney being empty, sexual and oppressive dreams, nocturnal emissions, premature ejaculation, cramp and paralysis of foot, red or white vaginal discharge, amenorrhoea, dysmenorrhoea, kidney weak, pain in loins, haemorrhoids, haematuria, face yellow-black, asthma.

Bladder 24

QI HAI YU   SEA OF QI YU

Extra associated point of upper lumbar region

Pain in loins, periumbilical pain, haemorrhoids, intestinal spasm, hypertension, gonorrhoea.

Bladder 25

DA CHANG YU   LARGE INTESTINE YU

Associated point of large intestine

Borborygmi, pain around umbilicus, diarrhoea, dry large intestine?, symptoms not changed by food or drink, pain in small intestine, loins cold and painful, weak legs, little urine, urethritis, dysuria, constipated, spasm of lumbar muscles.

Bladder 26

GUAN YUAN YU   GATE ORIGIN YU

Extra associated point of lower lumbar region

Pain in loins, passes little urine, abdomen swollen and tight, generalised disease of bowels, diarrhoea, emaciated, weakness after influenza, uterine spasm, lumbago, sciatica.

Bladder 27

XIAO CHANG YU   SMALL INTESTINE YU

Associated point of small intestine

Colitis, enteritis, diarrhoea, blood in stools, metritis, leucorrhoea, gonorrhoea, haemorrhoids, sacral pain, feet swollen.

Bladder 28

PANG GUANG YU   BLADDER YU

Associated point of bladder

Dysuria, haematuria, cystitis, urine dark yellow, lumbago, cramp in calves, abdominal pain, pain in lower leg, weakness of lower leg, head cold, metritis, poor circulation in young women.

Bladder 29

ZHONG LÜ YU   MIDDLE OF BACK YU

Extra associated point of sacrum

Kidneys weak, no perspiration, lumbago, back stiff, sciatica, dysentery with red and white flecks in motion, hernia, enterocolitis, abdominal pain.

Bladder 30

BAI HUAN YU   WHITE CIRCLE YU

Extra associated point of anal sphincter

Urine dark yellow or red, spermatorrhoea, amenorrhoea, metritis, incontinence of urine and faeces, spasm of anus, dysuria, lumbago and sacral pain, sciatica, quadriplegia.

Bladder 31

SHANG LIAO   UPPER BONE

Reunion B, G

Anuria, constipation, unable to become pregnant, prolapse of the uterus, red and white vaginal discharge, sciatica, lumbago, impotance, gonorrhoea, orchitis, epistaxis, a general point for genital diseases of both sexes

Bladder 32

CI LIAO   SECOND BONE

Pain and stiffness in loin and knee, swollen epigastrium, vomiting, dysuria, urine red, borborygmi, diarrhoea, red and white vaginal discharge, inflammation of scrotum, sterility, irregular menstruation, uterine prolapse, a general point for genital diseases of both sexes.

Bladder 33

ZHONG LIAO   MIDDLE BONE

Reunion B, G

Anuria, constipation, vomiting, abdominal swelling, diarrhoea, sterility, red and white vaginal discharge, amenorrhoea, pain in middle of lumbar and sacral region, a general point for genital diseases of both sexes.

Bladder 34
XIA LIAO   LOWER BONE

Borborygmi, blood in stools, diarrhoea, acute pain in lower abdomen, constipation, anuria, lumbago, coccydynia, pain and coldness down back and inside of thigh, a general point for genital diseases of both sexes.

Bladder 35
HUI YANG   MEETING OF THE YANG

Diarrhoea, pain in anal region, blood in stools, haemorrhoids, anal discharge, perianal diseases, gonorrhoea, sciatica, impotence, a general point for genital diseases of both sexes.

Bladder 36
FU FEN   SUPPLEMENTARY DIVISION

? Reunion B, Si   Brachial neuralgia, spasm of shoulder, neck painful and stiff, intercostal neuralgia, bronchitis, 'Wind and Cold enters the pores of the skin'.

Bladder 37
PO HU   SOUL SHELTER

Lungs are empty, weary and paralysed, dyspnoea, 'upper Qi', bronchitis, acute pain of the shoulders, vomiting, similar effect to that of the associated point of the lung B13.

Bladder 38
GAO HUANG   THE VITALS DIAPHRAGM

Specialised point for haematopoiesis   Weak, emaciated, five types of weariness, anaemia, spermatorrhoea, 'upper Qi', vomiting, dyspnoea, dry phlegm, madness, night sweats, loss of memory, difficulty in speaking, haemoptysis.

Bladder 39
SHEN TANG   SPIRIT HALL

Dyspnoea, asthma, all types of cardiac disease, 'upper Qi', contracture of back and renal area, shivering.

Bladder 40
YI XI SIGHING GIGLING

Dyspnoea, epistaxis, pericarditis, brachial neuralgia, intercostal neuralgia, fever without perspiration, slight fever, headache, fainting, cannot see clearly, spasm of back and loins, anorexia, vomiting.

Bladder 41
GE GUAN DIAPHRAGM GATE

Gastric bleeding, enterocolitis, middle of chest feels full, vomiting, belching, neither food nor drink can be swallowed, back rigid and painful, hypersalivation, nausea, fear of cold, dark yellow urine.

Bladder 42
HUN MEN SOUL DOOR

Chest feels full and melancholic, pleurisy, neither food nor drink can be swallowed, borborygmi, periumbilical pain, poor digestion, urine red or yellow, rheumatism, syncope.

Bladder 43
YANG GANG YANG ESSENTIALS

Abdomen distended, flatulence, diarrhoea due to large intestinal disease, urine red, dysuria, body hot with yellow eyes, unable to swallow food or drink, rheumatism.

Bladder 44
YI SHE THOUGHT SHELTER

Abdominal distension and flatulence, diarrhoea, weary, rheumatism, unable to swallow food or drink, vomiting without stopping, eyes yellow, urine dark yellow, intercostal neuralgia, afraid of cold, very thirsty, the more one drinks the greater is the thirst, localised oedema.

Bladder 45
WEI CANG   STOMACH GRANARY
Abdomen distended, ascites, unable to swallow food or drink, vomiting, backache, localised oedema

Bladder 46
HUANG MEN   VITALS DOOR
Inflammation of breast, pain below heart, spasm of stomach, constipation.

Bladder 47
ZHI SHI   AMBITIOUS ROOM
Pain and swelling in penis, all genital diseases, dysuria, kidney weakness, vomiting, abdominal swelling, back and kidney area rigid and painful, spermatorrhoea.

Bladder 48
BAO HUANG   WOMB AND VITALS
Pain in lower abdomen, constipation, retention of urine, heavy feeling pressing downwards, dysuria, pain and stiffness in back and renal area, orchitis, gonorrhoea, metritis, haemorrhoids, urethritis.

Bladder 49
ZHI BIAN   FOLDING EDGE
Lumbar and sacral pain, sciatica, pain and heaviness of genitalia, gynaecological diseases, difficult urination, cystitis, haemorrhoids of all types.

Bladder 50
CHENG FU   RECEIVE AND SUPPORT
Haemorrhoids, constipated, rectal pain, lumbago, pain in back, sciatica, coccydynia, difficulty in urination, pain in penis, spermatorrhoea, gynaecological diseases.

Bladder 51

YIN MEN PROSPEROUS GATE

Pain in back and loins, sciatica, unable to move foot, unable to look up or down — i.e. bend, bleeding haemorrhoids, circulatory disturbance of the thighs.

Bladder 52

FU XI FLOATING ACCUMULATION

Unable to bend knee, muscular spasm of lateral side of thigh, muscular spasm of calf, lower abdomen hot and hard on pressure, cystitis, constipation, vomiting.

Bladder 53

WEI YANG COMMANDING YANG

Lower meeting point Ho of triple warmer

Abdominal distension, muscular spasm of calf, muscular spasm in general, pain in loins, urinary incontinence, unable to look up or down — i.e. bend, cannot bend knee, chest feels full, pain and swelling of armpit, epilepsy, fever, fainting.

Bladder 54

WEI ZHONG COMMANDING MIDDLE

Earth point
Category VI
Lower meeting point Ho of bladder

Lumbago with stiff neck, arthritis of knee, foot swollen, body feels heavy, night sweats due to weakness, epistaxis, diarrhoea with a lot of blood in the motion, bleeding haemorrhoids, madness, spasms in children, nervousness, hemiplegia, abdominal pain, shivering, loss of hair head and eyebrows, skin diseases in general.

Bladder 55

HE YANG UNITING YANG

Hernia, rheumatism, madness, fits in children, pain in loins and abdomen, heaviness and muscular spasm in knee and calf, orchitis, menorrhagia, leucorrhoea, vaginal spasm.

Bladder 56
CHENG JIN   SUPPORTING MUSCLES
Pain and heaviness in foot and calf, pain of the instep of foot, muscular cramps, haemorrhoids of all types, epistaxis, constipation.

Bladder 57
CHENG SHAN   SUPPORTING MOUNTAIN
Head feels hot, epistaxis, epilepsy, abdominal pain, anorexia, swollen and bleeding haemorrhoids, knee swollen and painful, swelling of feet, lumbago, muscular cramps, gonorrhoea.

Bladder 58
FEI YANG   FLYING HIGH

Luo point   Epilepsy, head and eyes feel dizzy, vertigo, weakness of legs, lumbago, sciatica, supraorbital neuralgia, haemorrhoids, constipation, cystitis, irritable bladder, nocturia, pain in hypochondrium.

Bladder 59
FU YANG   FOOT BONE YANG

Point of Yang qiao mo
Accumulation point
of Yang qiao mo
Rheumatism of ankle, cramp, unable to bend knee or ankle, head heavy and painful, unable to raise arms or legs, thigh swollen.

Bladder 60
KUN LUN   KUN LUN MOUNTAINS (NEAR TIBET)

Fire point
Category V
Convulsions in little children, lumbago, pain in thigh, sciatica, rheumatism of foot, foot swollen, headache, eyes dizzy, vertigo, epistaxis, brachial neuralgia, haemorrhoids, retained placenta, glandular diseases, dyspnoea.

Bladder 61
PU SHEN   OFFICIAL'S AIDE

Point of Yang qiao mo   Foot paralysed, weakness of legs, lumbago, muscular cramp in calf, pain in knee, madness, sees ghosts, faints easily, gonorrhoea.

Bladder 62

SHEN MO EXTENDED MERIDIAN

Master point of Yang qiao mo
Coupled point of Yin qiao mo
Point of Yang qiao mo

Madness, epilepsy, dizziness, post-concussion symptoms, skin feels as if it is electrified or has too much energy, tinnitus, pain in knee and foot, foot red and swollen, lumbago, sciatica, occipital neuralgia, tension headaches, spastic conditions of uterus.

The symptoms of many diseases of the spinal cord can be helped, though not cured, in the early stages of the disease, by this point.

Bladder 63

JIN MEN GOLDEN DOOR

Accumulation point
Point of Yang wei mo

Headache, shaking of head with open mouth in children, convulsions in children, tinnitus, pain in knee and lower leg, lower abdominal pain, vomiting.

Bladder 64

JING GU CAPITAL BONE

Category IV
Source point

Lumbago, sciatica, stiff neck, torticollis, dyspnoea, pneumonitis, headache, epistaxis, epilepsy, madness, cerebral congestion, cardiac disease, inner canthus of eye is red, white membrane covers eye, dim vision, does not eat or drink.

Bladder 65

SHU GU BIND THE BONE

Wood point
Category III
Point of sedation

Enterocolitis, diarrhoea, fever, dislikes wind and cold, madness, headache, vertigo, inner canthus of eye red and painful, deafness, neck rigid, lumbago, sciatica, all types of haemorrhoids, all types of abscess.

Bladder 66

TONG GU PENETRATING THE VALLEY

Water point of Yang water meridian
Category II

Headache, vertigo, fear, stiff neck, epistaxis, rhinorrhoea, cannot see clearly, indigestion, gastritis, chest full, symptoms not altered by food or drink.

Bladder 67

ZHI YIN   EXTREMITY OF YIN

Metal point
Category I
Point of tonification
Point of exit

Head heavy, nose blocked, pain in eye, eye covered by membrane, intercostal neuralgia, fever without perspiration, difficulty in urination, effective in early prostatic hypertrophy, spermatorrhoea, 'old man's gait'. Be careful when using this point in a patient who easily gets supraorbital or occipital neuralgia.

Kidney

Kidney 1
YONG QUAN   BUBBLING SPRING

Wood point
Category I
Point of sedation (main)
Point of entry

Fainting with cold limbs, dumbness, prone to fear, madness or epilepsy, disturbed viscera (Zang-solid organs), alarm in children, paralysis (central Feng), pain in head and nape of neck, pain in throat and inability to swallow, throat numb, bleeding from nose, body painful and stiff, throat dry, great thirst, pain in small intestine, loins painful, hot disease spreading from loins around the body causing pain, pain in toes so that patient cannot wear shoes, stomach painful, loss of appetite, 'feet and heart hot', jaundice, chest and ribs full, eyes dizzy, vertigo, coughing, haemoptysis, dyspnoea, constipation, retention of urine, measles, hypertension, hypertensive encephalopathy, head feels congested with red face—looks like a beetroot.

Kidney 2
RAN GU   BLAZING VALLEY

Fire point
Category II
Point of sedation
(secondary)

Interior of throat swollen, throat numb, distension of lower abdomen, pain in chest, diarrhoea, dysentery, sharp pains in stomach, coughing blood, pain in legs and feet, oedema of feet, cold-damp feet, spermatorrhoea, impotence, irregular menstruation, pruritis vulvae, menorrhagia, prolapse of uterus, excessive eructation in children, night sweats.

Kidney 3
ZHAO HAI   SHINING SEA

Master point of Yin
qiao mo

Throat dry, four limbs weary, sadness, stage fright, madness or epilepsy at night, hemiplegia, lower abdomen painful, irregular menstruation, leucorrhoea, prolapse of uterus, pruritis vulvae, involuntary erections, gonorrhoea,

Coupled point of Ren mo	constipation, insomnia, sees stars and spots when he looks into the distance, asthma, neuralgia in arm and hand, headaches, migraine.
Point of Yin qiao mo	

Kidney 4
SHUI QUAN   WATER SPRING

Accumulation point Vision blurred, cannot see in the distance, myopia, periods do not come or when they come patient has much pain in abdomen, a few days before menstruation cries depressed anxious and nervous, abdominal pain, prolapse of uterus, frequent micturition, impotence.

Kidney 5
DA ZHONG   BIG BELL

Luo point Base of spine stiff and painful, heel swollen and painful, constipation, mouth hot, tongue dry, chest swollen, asthmatic breathing, haemoptysis, throat blocked and unable to swallow, noise in throat, patient fond of lying down, mental stupidity, prone to fear and unhappiness, wishes to remain at home, gonorrhoea, uterine spasm, dislikes the cold, vomits whatever he eats, stage fright, inferiority complex, nocturnal enuresis in children.

Kidney 6
TAI XI   BIGGER STREAM

Earth point
Category III & IV
Source

Coughing, coughing glutinous sputum, sharp pains in heart, urine dark yellow, defaecation difficult, fever without perspiration, fond of sleeping, throat swollen, haemoptysis, impotence, irregular periods, toothache, sores on both legs, heel swollen and painful, legs cold after a fever, spasm of diaphragm, anorexia, mammary pain, hand frozen.

Kidney 7
FU LIU   RETURNING CURRENT

Metal point
Category V

Abdomen distended like a drum, four limbs swollen, ascites, oedema, constant sweating, no sweating, hiccough, constipation, flatulence, dysentery,

Point of tonification

retention of urine, diabetes, spermatorrhoea, extreme fatigue, epistaxis, indigestion, haemorrhoids, pain in loins and back, cannot bear to move, vision dim, prone to anger and ceaseless talking, tongue dry, feet cold, feet paralysed, paralysis in children, myelitis, gonorrhoea, orchitis.

Kidney 8

JIAO XIN   EXCHANGE LETTERS

Point of Yin qiao mo
Accumulation point of
Yin qiao mo

Menorrhagia, irregular periods, amenorrhoea, red and white vaginal discharge, prolapse of uterus, loins thighs and legs painful, gonorrhoea, dysuria, orchitis, constipation, dysentery with pus and blood, perspires at night, one sided abdominal pain.

Kidney 9

ZHU BIN   BUILDING BANK

Point of Yin wei mo
Accumulation point of
Yin qiao mo

Legs weak, feet painful, insanity, swollen tongue, suddenly sticks out tongue, vomits mucus, muscular spasms in calf of leg, toxaemia of pregnancy with spasm of the lower abdominal muscles, no milk. According to Soulié de Morant, if this point is stimulated at the third and preferably also at the sixth month of pregnancy the infant when born will be healthier than normal, having a greater vitality and resistance to disease.

Kidney 10

YIN GU   YIN VALLEY

Water point of Yin
water meridian
Category VI

Pain in thighs, knees painful and cannot be flexed especially inner side, micturition difficult, abdomen and genitalia painful, abdominal pain radiating to umbilicus, abdomen distended like a drum, impotent, scrotum damp and itchy, pain radiating to genitalia on micturition, dysuria, urine dark yellow, incessant vaginal discharge, metrorrhagia, pruritis vulvae, hypersalivation.

Kidney 11

HENG GU   TRANSVERSE BONE (PUBIS)

Point of Chong mo

Abdomen swollen, lower abdomen painful, dysuria, five types of urethritis, vaginal prolapse, spermatorrhoea, not enough spermatozoa, penis and scrotum painful, amenorrhoea, eyes red and painful beginning in the inner corner of the eye, keratitis, lack of energy Yin due to abdominal pain, pain in renal area, cannot stand for a long time.

Kidney 12
DA HE   BIG BRIGHTNESS

Shokanten of greater
Yang
Point of Chong mo

Lower abdomen extremely swollen and painful, spermatorrhoea, pain in penis, vaginismus, frigidity, woman unable to conceive, chronic vaginitis, red vaginal discharge, eyes red and painful beginning at the inner corner of the eyes, cystitis, retention of urine, lumbago.

Kidney 13
QI XUE   QI HOLE

Confluence of vital
energy
This point is also called
'the door of infants'
Point of Chong mo

Infertility in women, irregular periods, Qi from upper abdomen attacks ribs and causes pain, Qi rushing madly up and down causing pain in loins, eyes red and painful beginning at the inner corners of the eyes, incessant diarrhoea, spermatorrhoea, impotence, pain in penis, paralysis of bladder.

Kidney 14
SI MAN   FOUR FULL

Point of Chong mo
This point is also called
'the palace of bone
marrow'

Hernia below the navel, abundant stools, indigestion, cutting pain below the navel, shivering with cold, spermatorrhoea, menorrhagia, irregular periods, dysmenorrhoea, urinary incontinence, Qi attacks ribs and causes pain, inner corner of eye red and painful.

Kidney 15
ZHONG ZHU   MIDDLE INJECTION

Point of Chong mo

Heat in upper abdomen, constipation, colitis, urinary incontinence, irregular periods, salpingitis, oophoritis, pain in loins and abdomen, inner corner of eyes red and painful, loss of energy, head clasped in a vice, pain and swelling in the joints of the fingers.

Kidney 16

HUANG YO   VITALS YU

Independent associated
point of intestines
Shokanten of lesser Yin
Point of Chong mo

Abdomen swollen and full, cutting pain in abdomen, constipated, diarrhoea, spasm of stomach, borborygmi, jaundice, eyes red and painful beginning at the inner corner of the eyes, five types of urethritis, spasm of the neck of the bladder, vaginismus.

Kidney 17

SHANG QU   MERCHANT'S TUNE

Point of Chong mo

Abdomen painful, cutting pain when abdomen full, no appetite, constipation or diarrhoea, gastric spasm, hyperacidity, anorexia, jaundice, congestion of eyes, dislikes living, sad, impatient, uterine spasm.

Kidney 18

SHI GUAN   STONE GATE

Point of Chong mo

Asthmatic breathing, hiccoughs, spleen and stomach empty and cold, anorexia, food and drink not digested, vomits food, sialorrhoea, bad blood in organs (Zang-solid organs) of women, unbearable pain in abdomen, constipation, eyes red and painful from inner corner of eyes, gonorrhoea, sterility, congestion and spasm of uterus, urine dark yellow, stiffness of vertebral column, 'upper Qi'.

Kidney 19

YIN DU   GHOST'S CAPITAL

Shokanten absolute Yin
—according to
Yosio Manaka
Point of Chong mo

Humming noise in adbomen, abdomen distended, abdominal pain, gastritis, duodenal or gastric ulcer, region below the heart distressed and melancholic, borborygmi, vomiting, flatulence, asthmatic breathing, rebellious Qi attacks ribs, eyes red and painful starting from the inner canthus, jaundice, 'upper Qi'.

Kidney 20

TONG GU (FU)   PENETRATING VALLEY (ABDOMEN)

Point of Chong mo

Dry mouth, dumbness, yawning, pain in ribs, pulmonary emphysema, dyspnoea, diarrhoea, food and drink not digested, acute and chronic gastritis, duodenal or gastric ulcer, stomach distended, diarrhoea, congestion of the eyes, rhinorrhoea, shaking with fright, stiff neck.

Kidney 21

YOU MEN   GATE OF HADES — THE PYLORUS

Shonkanten lesser Yang
— according to
Yosio Manaka
Point of Chong mo

Whole of chest painful, intercostal neuralgia, bronchitis, region below heart melancholic and full, pain on swallowing, no appetite, vomits mucus, upper abdomen swollen and full, diarrhoea containing blood, gastric or duodenal ulcer, jaundice, vomiting of pregnancy, amnesia, milk from breast does not come out, ulcer in breast, breast abscess, eyes red and painful starting from inner canthus, feeling of energy that rises.

Kidney 22

BU LANG   WALKING CORRIDOR

Point of exit

Chest and ribs full, dyspnoea, coughing, asthmatic, cannot raise arms, nose blocked, partial anosmia, vomiting, anorexia, oesophageal spasm, spasm of abdominis rectus, lack of energy, atony of large intestine, inflammation of breast.

Kidney 23

SHEN FENG   SPIRIT SEAL

Coughing, chest full, cannot breathe, bronchitis, ulcer of breast, tumour of breast, continually hot and cold, vomiting, anorexia, anosmia, spasm of rectus abdominis, angina pectoris, Judo knock-out point, tinnitus due to congestion, congestion of nose, hot flushes.

Kidney 24

LING XU   SPIRIT BURIAL-GROUND

Chest and diaphragm full and painful, incessant coughing, dyspnoea, bronchitis, pleurisy, vomiting, chest melancholia, anorexia, anxious, suspicious, amnesia, angina of effort, neuralgia of forearm, nose blocked, ozena, insomnia.

Kidney 25
SHEN ZANG   SPIRIT STORE
Chest and ribs full, coughing and unable to breathe, pulmonary congestion, bronchitis, vomiting, anorexia, stomach distended at midnight, insomia due to worry, does not wish to live, poor hearing.

Kidney 26
YU ZHONG   AMIDST ELEGANCE
Coughing, asthmatic breathing, intercostal neuralgia, unable to eat, chest and ribs full, bronchitis, ulcer of breast, excessive perspiration at night, easily becomes bad tempered, quick temperament, cerebral congestion, pruritis of ears, weakness of vocal cords, irritable cough, spits too much, palpitations, weight on chest, cold hands and feet, spasm of oesophagus and stomach, sialorrhea.

Kidney 27
YU FU   YU MANSION

Last point Coughing, chest full, cannot breathe, chest painful, chronic asthma, vomiting, anorexia, abdominal distension, oesophageal spasm, painful tongue, sensation that energy rises to top of body, jumps at sudden noises, irritable, headache due to excessive mental strain, pre-menstrual pain and tension, rhinophyma, brachial neuralgia.

Pericardium

(Envelope of the Heart or Circulation—Sex)

Circulation—Sex 1

TIAN CHI   HEAVENLY POND

Point of entry
Meeting point absolute
Yin
Point 'Window of the
sky'
? Reunion Cx, T

Fever without perspiration but with headache, chest-diaphragm distressed and melancholic, ribs painful, swelling under armpit, adenitis under arm, insufficient milk, mammary pain, cerebral congestion, paralysis of four limbs, foggy vision.

Circulation—Sex 2

TIAN QUAN   HEAVENLY SPRING

Cardiac pain, palpitations due to fear, chest-diaphragm full and painful, coughing, pulmonary congestion, bronchitis, chest and back swollen and inside of arm painful, anorexia, vomiting, fear of wind and cold, does not see clearly.

Circulation—Sex 3

QU ZE   CROOKED MARSH

Water point
Category VI

Body hot, very thirsty, dry mouth, rebellious Qi, stomach painful, vomiting, diarrhoea, arms trembling and painful, cholera, measles, perspiration of head and neck, chorea, myocarditis, sterility, neuralgia of upper arm, hemiplegia.

Circulation—Sex 4

XI MEN   ACCUMULATION DOOR

Accumulation point

Heart and chest painful, myocarditis, haemoptysis, epistaxis, nausea, haemorrhoids, weakness of tissues which bruise easily, spirit (heart) Qi insufficient, lack of energy, fear of surroundings and people, poor memory, neuralgia down middle of forearm and hand.

Circulation—Sex 5

JIAN SHI   THE INTERMEDIARY

Metal point
Category V
Group Luo point of
three upper Yin

Cardiac pain, carditis, heart suspended as though hungry, vomiting, cholera, malaria, gastritis, armpits swollen, cramp in elbow, palms of hands warm, insanity, fright in children, irregular periods, vaginal discharge, amenorrhoea, organs (Zang-solid organs) disordered, aphonia, pharyngitis, fear of wind and cold, hypertensive encephalopathy, neurasthenia, as if possessed of a devil.

Circulation—Sex 6

NEI GUAN   INNER GATE

Luo point
General Luo point
Master point Yin wei mo
Coupled point of Chong
mo

Headache, insomnia, dizziness, palpitation of heart, epilepsy, madness, easily frightened, swelling under armpits, cramp of elbow, cardiac pain, vomiting, middle regions blocked full and swollen, spleen and stomach not harmonised, stomach very painful, gastritis, enteritis, swelling of abdomen, diarrhoea, hiccoughs, coughing, depleted and weary, summer-heat diseases, rheumatism of foot, jaundice, irregular periods, post-partum bleeding and dizziness, spermatorrhoea, nearly pulseless.

Circulation—Sex 7

DA LING   BIG MOUND

Earth point
Category III & IV
Point of sedation
Source

Body hot, head painful, short of breath, chest and ribs painful, fever without perspiration, throat numb, ulcer of breast, arm cramp, armpits swollen, incessant laughter, prone to sadness, weariness and fear, mad speech and unhappiness, summer-heat diseases, ulcers of intestines, eyes red and painful, organs (Zang-solid organs) disordered, insanity, nerves weak.

Circulation—Sex 8

LAO GONG   LABOUR PALACE

Fire point of Ministerial
Yin fire meridian
Category II
Point of exit

Anger, incessant sadness or laughter, fever without perspiration, stomach painful, indigestion, blood in urine and stools, haemorrhoids, epistaxis, jaundice, very thirsty, pyorrhoea alveolaris, organs (Zang-solid organs) disordered, sensation that energy rises to top of body, writers' cramp, contracture of palmar aponeurosis.

Circulation—Sex 9

ZHONG CHONG   MIDDLE RUSHING

Wood point
Category I
Point of tonification
Last point

Fainting, delirium, unconsciousness, poor memory, severe fright, fevers with distress and melancholy but no sweating, palms of hands hot, body like fire, tongue rigid, stomach painful, temperature, vomiting and diarrhoea, all Yang diseases with fever, hyper or hypotension, cerebral congestion.

Triple Warmer

Triple Warmer 1

GUAN CHONG   GATE RUSHING

Metal point
Category I
Point of entry

Headache, throat numb, tongue curled up, dry mouth, vomiting, anorexia, pyrexia, cholera, summer-heat diseases, malaria, film over eyes, blurred vision, forearm painful and unable to raise.

Triple Warmer 2

YE MEN   FLUID DOOR

Water point
Category II

Hand and arm red and swollen, fingers cramped, forearm painful, all limbs icy cold, dizziness, slight deafness, tinnitus, headaches, eyes red swollen and painful, toothache, gingivitis, pharyngitis, malaria, wandering mind.

Triple Warmer 3

ZHONG ZHU   MIDDLE ISLET

Wood point
Category III
Point of tonification

Forearm and elbow painful, fingers cannot grasp objects tightly, fever without sweating, malaria, intermittent fevers, headache, vertigo, dizziness, tinnitus, slight deafness, film over eyes, pharyngitis, pain middle of back.

Triple Warmer 4

YANG CHI   YANG POND

Category IV
Source

Wrist painful and weak, wrist red and swollen, cannot be flexed or extended, hand and wrist bent, unable to grasp objects, forearm and elbow painful, brachial neuralgia, unable to raise arm, facial spasm, diabetes, mouth dry, melancholy, intermittent fever, shivering.

Triple Warmer 5

WAI GUAN   OUTER GATE

Luo point
General Luo point
Master point of Yang
wei mo
Coupled point of Dai mo

Forearm and elbow cannot be flexed, fingers painful and unable to grasp objects, muscles and bones of upper limb painful, rheumatism in general, slight deafness, epistaxis, toothache, hypertension, headache, pain in chest and ribs, cold, influenza, coughing, fever in general, summer-heat diseases, cholera, intestinal ulcers, infantile paralysis, violent fear, retained placenta.

Triple Warmer 6

ZHI GOU   BRANCH DITCH

Fire point of Ministerial
Yang fire meridian
Category V

Fevers without sweating, cholera, shoulder arms loin and back painful, rheumatism in general, ribs painful, pneumonia, pleurisy, chest-diaphragm troubled and melancholic, chest knotted, vomiting, difficulty in defaecation, limbs swollen and puffy, bleeding and fainting after childbirth, amenorrhoea, dumbness, lockjaw, eczema, cardiac pain.

Triple Warmer 7

HUI ZONG   MEETING ORIGIN

Accumulation point

Qi blocked up, epilepsy, nervous trembling, agitation, involuntary movement of fingers and arm, partial deafness, skin and flesh painful, dyspnoea.

Triple Warmer 8

SAN YANG LUO   THREE YANG LUO

Group Luo point of the
three upper Yang

Forearm and elbow painful and unable to raise, sleepiness, body does not wish to move, deafness, eye diseases, toothache, painful loins.

Triple Warmer 9

SI DU   FOUR GUTTERS

Forearm and elbow-joint painful, deafness, tinnitus, pharyngitis, toothache.

Triple Warmer 10

TIAN JING   HEAVENLY WELL

Earth point
Category VI
Point of sedation
Upper meeting point Ho
of triple warmer

Elbow and shoulder painful, unable to grasp objects, lumbago, cannot lie down, pain behind ear, tonsillitis, cervical adenitis, throat numb, cannot speak, jaw swollen and painful, outer corners of eyes red and swollen, one sided headache, tinnitus, partial deafness, heart and chest painful, coughing, bronchitis, dislikes food, insanity, excessive perspiration.

Triple Warmer 11

QING LENG YUAN   PURE COLD ABYSS

Elbow arm shoulder and back painful, cannot bend or stretch arm, cannot bear to wear clothes, headache, tinnitus, eyes yellow, ribs painful.

Triple Warmer 12

XIAO LUO   THAWING LUO RIVER

Arms and back swollen and painful, neck stiff, cervical adenitis, ulcers on arms, head dizzy, vertigo, occipital neuralgia.

Triple Warmer 13

NAO HUI   SHOULDER MEETING

Reunion T, Li
? Point of Yang wei mo

Arms painful and cannot be raised, elbow and forearm painful, difficult to flex or extend arm, shoulders and back painful, arm-pits very painful, goitre.

Triple Warmer 14

JIAN LIAO   SHOULDER BONE

Shoulder and arm painful and cannot move.

Triple Warmer 15

TIAN LIAO   HEAVENLY BONE

? Reunion T, G   Shoulder and back painful, arm and elbow painful and cannot be raised, neck

Point of Yang wei mo   stiff, pain in centre of clavicle, chest troubled and melancholic, absence of perspiration.

Triple Warmer 16
TIAN YOU   WINDOW OF HEAVEN

Point 'Window of the sky'   Shoulder back and arms painful, neck stiff, cannot turn neck, hyperacusis, suddenly becomes deaf, headache due to Wind, lively dreams, face swollen, eyes painful, vision confused.

Triple Warmer 17
YI FENG   WIND SCREEN

Reunion T, G   Tinnitus, partial deafness, pain in ears, dumb, inside of ear damp and itchy, facial paralysis, facial spasm, trigeminal neuralgia, mouth tightly clenched, jaw swollen, lower jaw painful, toothache, both sides of throat swollen, cervical adenitis, mumps.

Triple Warmer 18
QI MAI   FEEDING MERIDIANS

Headache, tinnitus, partial deafness, blurred vision, fits in children, epilepsy, convulsions, fear, vomiting, diarrhoea.

Triple Warmer 19
LU XI   SKULL REST

Body hot, head heavy, fits in small children, vomiting in children, convulsions, partial deafness, tinnitus, retinal haemorrhage, vomiting mucus and saliva, dyspnoea, ribs painful at sides, cannot turn body.

Triple Warmer 20
JIAO SUN   ANGLE OF THE EAR

Reunion T, G, ? Si,   Lobe of ear red and swollen, lips rigid, difficulty in chewing, gums swollen, optic nerve inflamed, film over eyes, exophthalmos, retinal haemorrhage.

Triple Warmer 21

ER MEN   EAR DOOR

Partial deafness, dumb, tinnitus, inside of ear painful, otitis media, otorrhoea, sores in ear, toothache, gingivitis, lips stiff, epistaxis.

Triple Warmer 22

(ER) HE LIAO (EAR) HARMONY BONE

Point of exit
? Reunion T, Si, G

Headache, facial paralysis, facial spasm, tinnitus, otitis externa, convulsions, neck and jaw swollen, rhinitis, nasal polyp.

Triple Warmer 23

SI ZHU KONG   SILK BAMBOO HOLLOW

Headache, eyes red and swollen and painful, eyes twitch or blink separately, optic atrophy, vision blurred, tears flow in bright light, inflammation of eyes due to electric light, vomits mucus and saliva, madness.

Gall Bladder

Gall Bladder 1

ZHONG ZI LIAO   EYE BONE

Point of entry
Meeting point lesser
Yang
Reunion G, Si, T

Headache, colour blindness, night blindness, optic atrophy, outer corners of eyes red and painful, myopia, retinal haemorrhage, conjunctivitis, keratitis, weak eye sight, trigeminal neuralgia, mouth and eyes awry, pharyngitis.

Gall Bladder 2

TING HUI   HEARING MEETING

Deafness and dumbness, pain inside ears, tinnitus, otorrhoea, mouth awry, jaw swollen, dislocation of jaw, toothache, gingivitis, dislikes cold food and drink, hemiplegia, convulsions, sad.

Gall Bladder 3

SHANG GUAN   UPPER GATE

Reunion G, S   Dislikes cold and wind, mouth and eyes awry, trismus, tinnitus, deafness, vertigo, pain one side of head, toothache, glaucoma, dislikes bright light.

Gall Bladder 4

HAN YAN   JAW DETESTED

Reunion G, S, T   Feng in the head, pain one side of head, mouth and eyes awry, foggy vision, tinnitus, deafness, vertigo, toothache, frequent sneezing, convulsions in children, hemiplegia, epilepsy, rheumatism, pain in neck.

Gall Bladder 5

XUAN LU   SUSPENDED SKULL

Reunion G, S, T   Pain on one side of head, toothache, epistaxis, purulent nasal discharge, face red and painful, outer corners of eyes red and painful, body hot, no sweating, melancholy.

Gall Bladder 6

XUAN LI   SUSPENDED BALANCE

Reunion G, S, ? T   Fevers without perspiration, headache on one side, trigeminal neuralgia, face red and swollen, outer corner of eyes red swollen and painful, melancholy of heart, anorexia.

Gall Bladder 7

QU BIN   TWISTED HAIR ON THE TEMPLES

? Reunion G, B   Mouth and eyes awry, cheeks and jaws swollen and painful, trismus, neck stiff and painful and unable to turn, headache on one side, retinal haemorrhage, eye diseases in general.

Gall Bladder 8

SHUAI GU   LEADING VALLEY

Reunion G, B   Headache, top of head painful, headache due to Wind on one or both sides, vomiting, eye diseases, melancholy, inability to eat or drink, drunkenness.

Gall Bladder 9

TIAN CHONG   HEAVEN RUSHING

Reunion G, B   Headache, insanity, epilepsy, muscular contractures, toothache, gums swollen and painful.

Gall Bladder 10

FU BAI   FLOATING WHITE

Reunion G, B   Throat numb, coughing, chest melancholy, dyspnoea, tinnitus, deafness, toothache, neck swollen and painful, tonsillitis, unable to move shoulders and back.

Gall Bladder 11

(TOU) QIAO YIN   (HEAD) EXTREME YIN

Reunion G, B, T   Headache, neck and jaws painful, throat numb, bitter taste in mouth, tongue stiff, tinnitus, dizziness, eyes painful, stiffness of limbs, no perspiration.

Gall Bladder 12

WAN GU   FINAL BONE

Reunion G, B   Headache, Wind affecting the head, face and head swollen, insanity, epilepsy, legs without strength, mouth and eyes awry, facial paralysis, otitis media, deafness, neck painful, torticollis, gingivitis, insomnia, urine dark yellow or red.

Gall Bladder 13

BEN SHEN   ROOT SPIRIT

Point of Yang wei mo   Penetrating Wind, unconsciousness, eyes dizzy, vertigo, neck stiff and painful, cannot turn neck, insanity, epilepsy, spitting saliva, fear, madness.

Gall Bladder 14

YANG BAI   YANG WHITE

Reunion G, Li, T
Point of Yang wei mo   Eyes red and swollen and painful, eyes twitch, dislikes bright light, headache, facial spasm, trigeminal neuralgia, nausea.

Gall Bladder 15

(TOU) LIN QI   (HEAD) ABOVE THE TEARS

Point of Yang wei mo   Outer corners of eyes painful, film over eyes, excessive formation of tears, nose blocked, fear of wind and cold, occipital headache, syncope, cerebral haemorrhage, cerebral congestion.

Gall Bladder 16

MU CHUANG   EYE WINDOW

Point of Yang wei mo   Colour blindness, eyes suddenly red swollen and painful, face and eyes swollen and puffy, weak eyesight, hazy vision, headache, dizziness, vertigo, fever without perspiration.

Gall Bladder 17

ZHENG YING   UPRIGHT YING

Point of Yang wei mo   Head and neck painful, toothache, lips stiff, gingivitis, vomiting, dizziness, dislikes hearing men's voices, weak eyesight.

Gall Bladder 18

CHENG LING   RECEIVING SPIRIT

Point of Yang wei mo   Headache, dislikes wind and cold, dyspnoea, epistaxis, nose blocked.

Gall Bladder 19

NAO KONG   BRAIN HOLLOW

Point of Yang wei mo   Headache, dizziness, unable to open eyes because of headache, photophobia, palpitations, dyspnoea, body hot, general weakness, neck stiff and cannot turn.

Gall Bladder 20

FENG CHI   WIND POND

Reunion G, T
Supposedly vaso-
sympathetic
Point of Yang wei mo
and probably Yang
qiao mo

Alternately hot and cold, sweatless fevers, colds, summer-heat diseases, migraine, headache, nervous debility, hemiplegia, cerebral haemorrhage, eyes dizzy, foggy vision, excessive formation of tears, eyes both dull, wind causes eyes to water, inner canthus red and painful, night blindness? retinal haemorrhage, optic atrophy, epistaxis, nose blocked, rhinorrhoea, inflammation of eye due to electric light, tinnitus, partial deafness, spine painful, rheumatism, stiff neck, painful shoulder, urticaria, poisoning.

Gall Bladder 21

JIAN JING   SHOULDER WELL

Reunion G, T
Point of Yang wei mo

Rheumatism, neck stiff, unable to turn neck, shoulder and back painful, arm painful, unable to raise hands to head, hemiplegia, cerebral congestion, vertigo, Qi blocked, phlegm rises, cannot speak, cervical adenitis, ulcers, boils, sores, retained placenta, post-partum haemorrhage, premature labour or miscarriage with cold limbs, breast abscess.

Gall Bladder 22

YUAN YE   ARMPIT ABYSS

Chest full, feeling of weakness in chest, pleurisy, intercostal neuralgia, cannot raise arms, goitre.

Gall Bladder 23

CHE JIN   FLANK MUSCLE

Alarm point
(secondary)

Chest very full preventing sleep, asthmatic respiration, cannot sleep well due to respiratory trouble, nervous depression, cannot speak clearly, vomiting stale fluid, swallowing stale saliva, warmth in the lower abdomen.

Gall Bladder 24

RI YUE   SUN AND MOON

Alarm point (main)
Reunion G, Sp
Point of Yang wei mo

Ribs painful, kidney Qi rushes against heart, vomiting, swallowing stale saliva, pain on swallowing, hiccoughs, frequent sighing, does not speak clearly, liver diseases, warmth in lower abdomen, spasms in limbs.

Gall Bladder 25

JING MEN   CAPITAL DOOR

Alarm point of kidney

Loins painful, cannot bend down, pain in hip joint, lumbago, pain back and shoulder, cannot remain standing a long time, abdomen distended, diarrhoea especially in a frightened person, borborygmi, asthma, dysuria, urine dark yellow.

Gall Bladder 26

DAI MO   DAI MO   (WAISTBAND EXTRA MERIDIAN)

Special for gynaeco-
logical diseases
Point of Dai mo

Lower abdomen painful, interior of body feels anxious, posterior part of body feels heavy, irregular menstruation, dysmenorrhoea, red or white vaginal discharge, vaginal prolapse, lower abdominal pain, false urge to go to stool in women due to pelvic pressure, loins as though 'seated in water'.

Gall Bladder 27

WU SHU   FIVE PIVOTS

Point of Dai mo

Loins and back painful, uterine spasm, red or white vaginal discharge, constipation, intestinal tumour? false call to stool in a woman, orchitis.

Gall Bladder 28

WEI DAO   BINDING PATH

Point of Dai mo   Loins and legs painful, lumbago, oedema, ascites, vomiting, anorexia, inflammation of intestines, nephritis, orchitis.

Gall Bladder 29

JU LIAO   DWELLING BONE

Point of Yang qiao mo   Paralysis, loins and lower abdomen painful, dysmenorrhoea, irregular periods, leucorrhoea, cystitis, nephritis, orchitis, diseases of upper limbs, pain radiating from shoulder to chest.

Gall Bladder 30

HUAN TIAO   JUMPING CIRCLE

Reunion G, B.   Half of body uncoordinated, paralysis, epilepsy, loins and spine painful, loins and thighs painful, buttocks over ischium painful, sciatica, unable to turn, rheumatism in general, pain in knee, influenza, nervous exhaustion.

Gall Bladder 31

FENG SHI   WIND MARKET

Paralysis, paralysis of lower limbs, paralysis in children, weakness of the legs in general, sciatica, generalised pruritis, sores.

Gall Bladder 32

ZHONG DU   MIDDLE DITCH

Half of body uncoordinated, sciatica, lumbago, loins and legs painful, weakness in general of the legs, muscular spasms in legs, passage point with three lower Yang.

Gall Bladder 33

(XI) YANG GUAN   (KNEE) YANG GATE

Knees red, swollen and painful, knee cannot be flexed or extended, loss of sensation in knee.

Gall Bladder 34

YANG LING QUAN   YANG MOUND SPRING

Earth point
Category VI
Lower meeting point Ho
of gall bladder
Specialised point for
muscles

Half body uncoordinated, lower limbs cold and numb, legs cold as though without blood, lumbago, sciatica, knees red swollen and painful, special point for the knee, neurasthenia, ribs painful, face swollen, pharyngitis, extreme fright, insanity, madness, constipation.

Gall Bladder 35

YANG JIAO   YANG CROSSING

Point of Yang wei mo
Accumulation point
Yang wei mo

Throat numb, chest full, dyspnoea, pleurisy, face swollen, and puffy, sciatica, weakness and neuralgia of peroneal muscles, weakness of legs, cold feet.

Gall Bladder 36

WAI QIU   OUTER MOUND

Accumulation point

Paralysis, muscular spasm in calves, beri-beri, neck painful, chest and ribs swollen and painful, dislikes wind and cold, insanity, madness.

Gall Bladder 37

GUANG MING   LIGHT BRIGHT

Luo point

Muscular pain in legs, cannot stand for long periods, paralysis of lower limbs, muscular spasm or neuralgia in calves, sweatless fevers, all eye diseases, becomes suddenly mad.

Gall Bladder 38

YANG FU   YANG SUPPORT

Fire point
Category V
Point of sedation

Paralysis, muscular spasm, vascular spasm, generalised arthralgia, generalised aches and pains, pain in chest and buttocks and knees extending to ankles, sciatica, loins as though sitting in water, corners of eyes painful, bitter taste in mouth, throat numb, cervical adenitis, goitre, likes to sigh, pasty skin, axillary and clavicular swellings.

Gall Bladder 39

XUAN ZHONG   SUSPENDED BELL

Group Luo point of
three lower yang
Specialised point for
bone marrow,
leucocytosis

Penetrating wind, cerebral haemorrhage, hands and feet uncoordinated, stomach and abdomen swollen and full, no appetite, acute appendicitis, diarrhoea, haemorrhoids, rheumatism, loins painful, beri-beri, lower part of leg painful, cannot rise after sitting down, Shang han with high fever which does not subside, throat numb, epistaxis, inside of nose dry, chorea, neurasthenia, madness, fear, bad temper.

Gall Bladder 40

QIU XU   GRAVE MOUND

Category IV
Source point

Chest and ribs painful, cannot breathe, swelling under arms, paralysis, cannot rise after sitting, pain in buttocks, lower limbs painful, muscular spasm, sciatica, heels red, heels swollen and painful, neck swollen, pain in lower abdomen, conjunctivitis.

Gall Bladder 41

(ZU) LIN QI   (FOOT) ABOVE TEARS

Wood point of Yang
wood meridian
Category III
Point of exit
Master point of Dai mo
Coupled point of Yang
wei mo

Lower part of legs and feet damp and swollen, rheumatic pains that move around, ribs full and painful, irregular menstruation, dysmenorrhoea, ulcers of the breast, axillary adenitis, vertigo, mastoid pain, intermittent fever, excessive perspiration.

Gall Bladder 42

DI WU HUI   EARTH FIVE MEETINGS

Extensor surface of foot red and swollen, ulcers of the breast, pain and swelling of axilla, eyes red and painful.

Gall Bladder 43

XIA XI   CHIVALROUS STREAM

Water point
Category II
Point of tonification

Extensor surface of foot red and swollen, spasm of the five toes, space between toes damp and rotten, four limbs swollen and puffy, ribs painful, pleurisy, jaw swollen, tinnitus, partial deafness, vertigo, sweatless fever, outer canthus red and swollen, cerebral congestion.

Gall Bladder 44

(ZU) QIAO YIN (FOOT) EXTREME YIN

Metal point
Category I
Last point

Headache, dreams of ghosts, heart troubled, eyes painful, ribs painful, cannot breathe, coughing, excessive sleep, insomnia, cannot raise arm, hands and feet hot, no perspiration, throat numb, tongue stiff, mouth dry, deafness.

Liver

Liver 1

XING JIAN COLUMN INBETWEEN

DA DUN BIG HEAP

Wood point of Yin
wood meridian
Category I
Point of entry

Frequency of micturition, incontinence of urine, one side of scrotum enlarged, pain in penis, gonorrhoea, vaginal prolapse, pruritis vulvae, menorrhagia, polymenorrhoea, abdominal pain, abdominal swelling, pain in
stomach, 'penetrating Wind', unconsciousness, fainting, appearance as though
dead, likes to sleep, headaches, excessive perspiration, lumbago.

Liver 2

XING JIAN COLUMN INBETWEEN

Fire point
Category II
Point of sedation

Headache, head dizzy, insomnia, angry easily, eyes red swollen and weepy,
throat dry and irritated, chest and ribs painful, coughing due to emptyness
and weariness, gastric pain, haematemesis, whole abdomen swollen, lower
abdomen swollen, retention of urine, excessive and ceaseless menstrual bleeding, loins painful, cannot bend, knees swollen and painful, dry and wet beri-
beri, inter-digital swelling, hysteria, madness, insanity, epilepsy, fits, convulsions in children, neurasthenia, carbuncle, ulcer or abscess of breast.

Liver 3

TAI CHONG BIGGER RUSHING

Earth point
Category III & IV
Source
Independent associated
point for spasms

Stomach painful, throat dry, nausea, vomiting, dry lips, chest and ribs full
and painful, cervical or axillary swelling, lower abdomen swollen, diarrhoea,
constipation, loins and lower abdomen painful, incontinence of urine,
urethritis, retracted scrotum, haematuria, constant uterine bleeding, pain in
front of internal malleolus, difficulty in walking, feet weak, spasms or cramp
of toes, face and eyes pale, does not see clearly.

Liver 4

ZHONG FENG   MIDDLE SEAL

Metal point
Category V
Swelling of abdomen, lower abdomen distended, eyes yellow with slight fever, jaundice, anorexia, feels ill after food, pain around body at level of navel, loins painful, feet and legs cold, muscular atony, spermatorrhoea, impotence, urethritis, pain in vagina.

Liver 5

LI GOU   INSECT DITCH

Luo point
Violent pain in abdomen, lower abdomen swollen, retention of urine, sudden pain in scrotum, menorrhagia, irregular periods, vaginal discharge, belching, throat feels obstructed, fear and nervousness, depression, dejection, cramp in back, cannot bend back, skin cold and aching, difficult to flex knee.

Liver 6

ZHONG DU   MIDDLE CAPITAL

Accumulation point
Lower abdominal pain, diarrhoea, large stools, feet weak withered and emaciated, cannot walk or stand, pain in knee, skin cold numb and painful, menorrhagia, pharyngitis.

Liver 7

XI GUAN   KNEE GATE

'Wind' rheumatism, pain in throat, inside of knee and patella painful, cannot bend knee.

Liver 8

QU QUAN   CROOKED SPRING

Water point
Category VI
Point of tonification
Fibroids, abdomen swollen, abdominal colic, irregular periods, vaginal prolapse, pruritis vulvae, pain in vagina and thighs, pain in penis, spermatorrhoea, dysuria, retention of urine, rectal discharge of thick blood, dysentery, knees painful with cramped muscles and inability to flex, knees and shins cold

and painful, lower abdominal pain extending to throat, epistaxis, madness, paraplegia.

Liver 9
YIN BAO   YIN WRAPPING
Loins and base of spine painful extending to lower abdomen, muscular spasm of loins and buttocks, dysuria, incontinence of urine, irregular periods, boils on both buttocks, fullness of chest.

Liver 10
(ZU) WU LI   (FOOT) FIVE MILE
Abdomen full, retention of urine, spermatorrhoea, scrotum damp and itching, helps perspiration and sleep.

Liver 11
YIN LIAN   YIN SCREEN
Women cease to bear children, irregular periods, leucorrhoea, pruritis vulvae.

Liver 12
JI MAI   QUICK PULSE
Penis painful, inside of buttocks or thighs painful.

Liver 13
ZHANG MEN   CHAPTER DOOR

Alarm point of spleen Centre reunion particular point of five Zang (solid) organs Shokanten of greater Yin Reunion Liv, G Point of Dai mo

Oedema, ascites, borborygmi, abdominal swelling, abdomen distended like a drum, food not digested, diarrhoea, stomach painful, flatulence, mouth dry, anorexia, over-eating, chest and ribs painful, ribs painful — cannot lie down, body hot — heart troubled, hypertension, stertorous respiration, loins painful — cannot turn over, jaundice, loss of weight with slightly yellow skin.

Liver 14

QI MEN   PERIOD DOOR

Point of alarm
Point of exit
Shokanten of absolute
Yin
Reunion Liv, Sp, ? G
Point of Yin wei mo

Chest-diaphragm distended, coughing, stertorous respiration, belching, vomiting sour fluid, food and drink do not descend, mouth dry, very thirsty, diarrhoea, abdomen hard, peritonitis, both sides of body painful, sharp pain in wrist, hypertension, difficult delivery, post partum troubles.

Conception Vessel

Conception Vessel 1

HUI YIN   MEETING OF YIN

General Luo point
Reunion Cv, Gv
Point of Chong mo

All diseases of perineal area, pruritis vulvae, excessive perspiration in perineal area, pain in vagina, outer part of vagina swollen and painful, prolapse of vagina, irregular periods, dysmenorrhoea, amenorrhoea in young women, spermatorrhoea, scrotum cold, penis painful and cold, pruritis ani, haemorrhoids, constipation with infrequent micturition, nocturnal perspiration that is not salty.

Conception Vessel 2

QU GU   CROOKED BONE

Reunion Cv, Liv

Lower abdomen swollen and full or extremely painful, retention of urine with overflow, incontinence of urine, cystitis, red or white vaginal discharge, gonorrhoea, vaginismus, metrorrhagia, menorrhagia, uterus does not reduce in size within normal period after delivery, spermatorrhoea, impotance, scrotum wet and itchy, lack of virility.

Conception Vessel 3

ZHONG JI   MIDDLE EXTREMITY

Alarm point of bladder
Reunion Cv, Sp, K, Liv

Lump below navel like upturned cup, fibroids, irregular periods, dysmenorrhoea, menorrhagia, excessive white vaginal discharge, pruritis vulvae, vaginal orifice swollen and painful, pain in vagina, prolapse of vagina, retained placenta, incessant discharge after confinement, impotence, spermatorrhoea, dysuria, haematuria, urinary incontinence, frequent micturition, fainting, general fatigue, ascites.

Conception Vessel 4
GUAN YUAN   GATE ORIGIN

Alarm point of small
intestine
Reunion Cv, Sp, K, Liv

Abdomen painful, dysentery, cholera, diarrhoea, prolapse of rectum, lines of pain around navel, abdomen swollen like a drum, fibroids below navel like upturned cup, dysuria, haematuria, urinary incontinence, spermatorrhoea, impotence, vaginal discharge, irregular menstruation, light periods of long duration, dysmenorrhoea, prolapse of vagina, pruritis vulvae, abdomen painful after confinement, incessant discharge after confinement, retained placenta, jaundice, hypertension, neurasthenia.

Conception Vessel 5
SHI MEN   STONE DOOR

Alarm point of triple
warmer — main
Centre of energy

Abdomen swollen painful and hard, colitis, incessant diarrhoea, pain in lower abdomen, haematemesis, periumbilical pain, ascites, food not digested, micturition infrequent, urinary diseases, menorrhagia, vaginal discharge. Original Qi of lower triple warmer in males and females of all ages empty and cold.

Conception Vessel 6
QI HAI   SEA OF QI

Centre of energy

Stomach painful, abdomen painful, periumbilical pain, cold and pain below navel, ascites, abdomen swollen like drum, fibroids and tumours in abdomen, swelling in abdomen which does not descend when pressed, hiccoughing, vomiting, constipated, haematuria, dysuria, Zang Qi empty and melancholy, true Qi deficient, chronic Qi diseases, body emaciated, emptyness, weariness, limbs weak, patient wishes to die, Yin diseases, limbs cold, menorrhagia, red and white vaginal discharge, amenorrhoea, irregular periods, dysmenorrhoea, incessant discharge after confinement, abdomen swollen after confinement, retained placenta, prolapse of vagina, spermatorrhoea, impotence, enuresis in children, hypertension, insomnia.

Conception Vessel 7

YIN JIAO   YIN CROSSING

Alarm point of triple warmer — lower Reunion Cv, Cx, T Point of Chong mo

Pain below navel, cold and pain around navel, abdomen full, abdomen hard and painful, sweating and pruritis of genitalia, urethritis, cannot urinate, sterility, menorrhagia, irregular periods, vaginal discharge, incessant discharge after confinement, fainting, post-partum madness, acute tonsillitis, epistaxis.

Conception Vessel 8

SHEN QUE   SPIRIT SHRINE

Incessant diarrhoea, ascites, abdomen swollen like drum, abdominal pain, periumbilical pain, abdomen empty, intestinal noises like sound of flowing water, rectal prolapse, penetrating Wind, fainting, unconsciousness, cerebral haemorrhage, incessant lactation.

Conception Vessel 9

SHUI FEN   WATER DIVISIONS

Reunion Cv, L

Water diseases, ascites, oedema, abdomen swollen like drum, stomach empty and swollen, anorexia, pain round body at level of navel, borborygmi, flatulence, a rushing up into the chest which causes inability to breathe, pain in renal area, fontanelles weak, epistaxis.

Conception Vessel 10

XIA WAN   LOWER CHANNEL

Reunion Cv, Sp

Abdomen painful, abdomen distended, vomiting, anorexia, tumour in abdomen (?), food not digested, gradual emaciation, abdomen swollen like a drum, stomach ache, gastritis, gastric spasm, dilation of stomach, haematuria.

Conception Vessel 11

JIAN LI   ESTABLISHED MILE

Abdomen swollen, abdomen painful, body swollen, stomach painful, spasms of lower abdomen, vomiting, anorexia, poor digestion, cardiac pain with sensation of energy that moves to upper part of body.

Conception Vessel 12

ZHONG WAN   MIDDLE CHANNEL

Alarm point of stomach and triple warmer — middle

Centre reunion particular point of five Fu (hollow) organs

Reunion Cv, Si, S, T, L, Cx, ? Liv

Abdomen painful, abdomen swollen, all gastric diseases, cholera, vomiting, swallowing sour saliva, vomiting sour matter, stomach pain, acute gastro-enteritis, food difficult to digest, abdomen swollen like drum, diarrhoea, constipation, intestinal abscess, prolapse of vagina, jaundice, insomnia, headache, palpitations of heart, chronic spleen Wind, ribs painful, hiccoughing, dyspnoea, hypertension, insanity, madness, paralysis, penetrating Wind, face numb and yellow.

Conception Vessel 13

SHANG WAN   UPPER CHANNEL

Reunion S, Si, L

Vomiting, food does not descend, abdomen swollen, abdomen painful, diarrhoea, Qi full, peritonitis, food not digested, pain in stomach, hard mass in abdomen like a dish, haematemesis, jaundice, hiccoughing, pleurisy, bronchitis, insanity, madness, fear, epilepsy, body hot and sweaty, cardiac pain with sensation of warmth.

Conception Vessel 14

JU QUE   GREAT SHRINE

Alarm point of heart

Coughing, Qi rises, chest full, dyspnoea, chest painful, cardiac pain, sour taste in mouth, vomits sour matter, vomiting, diarrhoea, abdomen swollen and very painful, jaundice, hiccoughs, acute gastro-enteritis, fainting, confusion and melancholy, insanity, madness, fear, forgetfulness, beri-beri.

Conception Vessel 15

JIU WEI   DOVE TAIL

Luo point

Centre reunion particular point of vital centres

Chest full, coughing, haemoptysis, throat numb, throat swollen — fluid does not descend, dyspnoea, hiccoughing, vomiting, gastric pain, palpitations, cardiac diseases, anti-smoking, insanity, hysteria, walks around wildly, cannot choose correct words, unilateral headache, loss of virility.

Conception Vessel 16

ZHONG TING   MIDDLE COURTYARD

Chest and ribs swollen and painful, dyspnoea, throat blocked — appears like a plum stone — tonsillitis, food does not descend, nausea, vomiting, vomiting milk by children.

Conception Vessel 17

SHAN ZHONG   PLATFORM MIDDLE

Alarm point of Cx
Alarm point of triple
warmer — upper
and ? of Cx
Centre reunion particular of breath energy
Sea of energy
Reunion Cv, Si, T, K, Cx
? L, ? H

Dyspnoea, lung abscess, coughing, all lung diseases, haematemesis, haemoptysis, heart and chest painful, anti-smoking, insufficient lactation, abdomen swollen like a drum.

Conception Vessel 18

YU TANG   JADE HALL

Chest painful, coughing, Qi rises, pleurisy, bronchitis, vomiting cold phlegm, chest full, cannot breathe, dyspnoea, cardiac pain, haemoptysis.

Conception Vessel 19

ZI GONG   PURPLE PALACE

Chest painful, coughing, dyspnoea, bronchitis, vomiting cold phlegm, both breasts swollen and painful cardiac pain, food and drink do not descend, vomiting food.

Conception Vessel 20

HUA GAI   SPLENDOUR COVERING

Sides of chest full and painful, coughing, Qi rises, dyspnoea, throat numb, glosillitis, throat swollen, unable to swallow liquids, anti-smoking, spasm of notttis, asthma.

Conception Vessel 21

XUAN JI   PEARL JADE

Sides of chest full and painful, coughing, dyspnoea, throat numb, throat swollen, tonsillitis, aerogastria, unable to swallow liquids.

Conception Vessel 22

TIAN TU   HEAVEN RUSHING

Point 'Window of the sky'
Point of Yin wei mo

Dyspnoea, dry cough, noise in throat like sound of a crane (bird), cardiac pain, Qi rebellious in chest, lung abscess, bronchitis, asthma, haemoptysis, throat swollen, sores in throat which prevent eating, dumbness, aphonia, oesophageal spasm, glottic spasm, stiff tongue, veins on underside of tongue congested, partial deafness, goitre, cervical adenitis, jaundice, vomiting, acute gastro-enteritis, falls asleep too easily, face red with sensation that energy rises to the upper part of body.

Conception Vessel 23

LIAN QUAN   SCREEN SPRING

Point of Yin wei mo

Tongue stiff, tongue loose, dribbles saliva, sores in mouth, veins under tongue swollen, difficulty in speaking, throat constricted, hacking cough, dyspnoea, bronchitis, deafness and dumbness, excessive thirst.

Conception Vessel 24

CHENG JIANG   RECEIVING FLUID

Reunion Cv, Li, S

Head and back of neck stiff and painful, half body uncoordinated, hemiplegia, mouth and eyes awry, trismus, face swollen, toothache, gingivitis, dental caries, excessive thirst, complete dumbness, insanity, fear.

Governing Vessel

Governing Vessel 1

CHANG QIANG   LONG STRENGTH

Luo point
General Luo point
Reunion Gv, G, K

Lower back painful, haemorrhoids, intestinal haemorrhage, haematemesis, rectal prolapse, wind in large intestine, extreme nervousness, convulsions, madness, micturition and defaecation difficult, diarrhoea, impotence, spermatorrhoea, pruritis vulvae.

Governing Vessel 2

YAO YU   LOINS YU POINT

Independent associated point of renal area

Loins and back stiff and painful, feet paralysed, haemorrhoids, irregular periods, malaria and other fevers, urine dark red.

Governing Vessel 3

(YAO) YANG GUAN (LOINS) YANG GATE

Lumbago, knees painful, cannot bend knees, spermatorrhoea, leucorrhoea, abdominal distension, diarrhoea, colitis.

Governing Vessel 4

MING MEN   GATE OF LIFE

Headache, body extremely hot, no perspiration, intermittent fevers, pain in lumbar region and abdomen together, lumbar pain, nervousness in children, convulsions, tinnitus, red or white vaginal discharge, impotence, spermatorrhoea, haemorrhoids, rectal prolapse, neurasthenia, insomnia, oedema, incontinence of urine.

Governing Vessel 5

XUAN SHU   SUSPENDED PIVOT

Loins and back stiff and painful, food not digested, epigastric discomfort, stools loose, frequency of micturition.

Governing Vessel 6

JI ZHONG   MIDDLE OF SPINE

Insanity, epilepsy, abdomen distended and full, anorexia, jaundice, stomach turns over, haematemesis, haemorrhoids, blood in stools, diarrhoea, prolapse of rectum.

Governing Vessel 7

ZHONG SHU   MIDDLE PIVOT

Pain in lower thoracic and lumbar region, stomach ache, deterioration in eyesight.

Governing Vessel 8

JIN SUO   CONTRACTED MUSCLE

Insanity, epilepsy, walking around madly, rolling of eyes, eyes fixed in an upward direction, cardiac pain, lower back extremely stiff, stomach ache.

Governing Vessel 9

ZHI YANG   EXTREME YANG

Loins and back painful, chest and back painful, shins aching, limbs weary and heavy, chest distended, dyspnoea, difficulty in speaking, stomach feels cold, cannot eat, jaundice, borborygmi, intermittent fevers.

Governing Vessel 10

LING TAI   SUPERNATURAL TOWER

Dyspnoea, asthma, bronchitis, pneumonia, insomnia—especially if caused by dyspnoea, loins and back painful.

Governing Vessel 11

SHEN DAO   SPIRIT PATH

Cardiac diseases in general, fever, dislikes cold, headache, intermittent fever, forgetfulness, nervousness, nervousness and insanity in children, convulsions, back rigid and painful.

Governing Vessel 12

SHEN ZHU   BODY PILLAR

Epilepsy, convulsions, extreme nervousness in children, body hot, suicidal, incoherent speech, madly walking around, loins and spine rigid and painful, rheumatic diseases, epistaxis.

Governing Vessel 13

TAO DAO   KILN PATH

Reunion Gv, B   Head heavy, eyes dizzy, vertigo, convulsions, depression, spine rigid, neck, shoulders and back painful, fever with dislike of cold, intermittent fevers, no sweating, inflammatory diseases of bones, numbness in children, amenorrhoea, urticaria.

Governing Vessel 14

DA ZHUI BIG HAMMER — VERTEBRA

Centre reunion general point of Yang Reunion of all Yang meridians including Gv   Headache, neck stiff and cannot turn, hysteria, wind diseases, rheumatic (Numb) diseases, paralysis, numbness in children, St. Vitus' Dance, neurasthenia, retinal haemorrhage, epistaxis, gingivitis, chest distended, hacking cough, loins and spine painful, intermittent fever, fever with dislike of cold, summer-heat diseases, vomiting, cholera, jaundice, urticaria.

Governing Vessel 15

YA MEN   DOOR OF DUMBNESS

Reunion Gv, B Point of Yang wei mo   Headache, neck stiff, spine rigid, epilepsy, convulsions, tongue moves slowly, cannot speak, swelling of sublingual area, complete or partial loss of voice, deafness and dumbness, epistaxis.

Governing Vessel 16

FENG FU   WIND MANSION

Point 'Window of sky'
Sea of bone marrow
Reunion Gv, B
Point of Yang wei mo

Headache, vertigo, epistaxis, nose blocked, throat swollen and painful, deafness and dumbness, neck stiff, cannot turn neck, toothache, hemiplegia, cerebral haemorrhage, tongue slow — cannot speak, walks around madly, eyes move wildly, suicidal, fear, colds, influenza.

Governing Vessel 17

NAO HU   BRAIN SHELTER

Reunion Gv, B

Eyes painful, cannot see long distances, head heavy, neck stiff and painful.

Governing Vessel 18

QIANG JIAN   STRENGTH INBETWEEN

Unbearable headaches, vertigo, vomiting, epilepsy, insomnia, depression, neck stiff — cannot turn, cardiac discomfort.

Governing Vessel 19

HOU DING   POSTERIOR SUMMIT

Headache, migraine, fear of wind and cold, head and neck stiff, vertigo, epilepsy, walks around madly, insomnia.

Governing Vessel 20

BAI HUI   HUNDRED MEETINGS

Centre reunion general point of Yang
Reunion Gv, B, ? Liv
Sea of bone marrow

Headache, penetrating Wind, vertigo, hemiplegia, cerebral haemorrhage, fainting with trismus, delirium, extreme nervousness, forgetfulness, frequent weeping, unable to choose words, madness, insanity, severe fright, hysteria, neurasthenia, eclampsia, menorrhagia, cardiac discomfort, tinnitus, partial deafness, nose blocked, anosmia, rectal prolapse, haemorrhoids, retention of urine, sterility in women, convulsions in children, stiff spine, heavy head.

Governing Vessel 21

QIAN DING   ANTERIOR SUMMIT

Headache, vertigo, extreme nervousness in children, convulsions, epilepsy, rhinorrhoea, nasal polyp, face red and swollen.

Governing Vessel 22

XIN HUI   SKULL MEETING

Vertigo, nervousness, eyes stare upwards, cannot recognise people, face swollen, face too red or pale, epistaxis, nose blocked, anosmia.

Governing Vessel 23

SHANG XING   UPPER STAR

Headache, eyes painful, cannot see far, nose blocked, nasal polyp, purulent rhinorrhoea, epistaxis, face red and swollen, fever without perspiration.

Governing Vessel 24

SHEN TING   SPIRIT COURTYARD

Reunion Gv, S, B   Violent headache, eyes weepy, eyes red swollen and painful, rhinorrhoea, eyes stare upwards and cannot recognise people, climbing to high place and singing, taking off clothes and walking, suddenly sticks tongue out, dyspnoea with thirst, vomiting.

Governing Vessel 24.5

YIN TANG   SEAL PALACE

Nervousness in children, headache, vertigo, eye diseases in general, nasal catarrh, nose blocked, trigeminal neuralgia, uterine bleeding after confinement, eclampsia, vomiting, diarrhoea.

Governing Vessel 25

SU LIAO   ELEMENT BONE

Nose blocked, nasal polyp, sores inside nose, bulbous nose from drinking excessive alcohol, epistaxis.

Governing Vessel 26

REN ZHONG MIDDLE OF THE MAN

Reunion Gv, Li, S Fainting, delirium, epilepsy, madness, hysteria, severe fright, Penetrating Wind, eclampsia, menorrhagia, bleeding and dizziness after confinement, oedema, excessive thirst, summer-heat diseases, lumbago, pain along vertebral column.

Governing Vessel 27

DUI DUAN EXTREME EXCHANGE

Fainting, delirium, epilepsy, hysteria, incessant epistaxis, lips stiff, toothache, gingivitis, tongue dry, excessive thirst, swelling of chin, urine yellow.

Governing Vessel 28

YIN JIAO GUM CROSSING

Reunion Gv, Cv Sores on face in children, gingivitis, excessive weeping, inner corners of eyes red itching and painful, white film over eyes, nose blocked, nasal polypus, cardiac pain, melancholic feeling in cardiac area.

Non Meridian Points

Head

SI SHEN CONG   FOUR SPIRIT ABILITY

*XH*1   Headache, dizziness, epilepsy.
(One Chinese inch in front, behind, to left and right of Gv 20.)

YIN TANG   SEAL PALACE

*XH*2   See Gv 24.5

TAI YANG   SUPREME YANG

*XH*3   Headache, head dizzy, neurasthenia, trigeminal neuralgia, optic nerve atrophy, retinal haemorrhage, eyes red swollen and painful, toothache.

NEI JING MING   INNER BRIGHT EYES

*XH*4   Conjunctivitis, optic nerve atrophy, retinal haemorrhage, various eye diseases.
(Medial corner of eye — middle of caruncle.)

Nose

NEI YING XIANG   INNER WELCOME FRAGRANCE

*XN*1   Severe headaches, severe pain in eyes, fevers.
(Inside ala of nose.)

SHANG YING XIANG   UPPER WELCOME FRAGRANCE

*XN*2   Headaches, nose blocked.

Mouth

JU QUAN   COLLECTED SPRING

*XM*1   Rigid tongue, dyspnoea, coughing.

XM2 left   JIN JIN   GOLDEN FLUID

YU YE   JADE FLUID
XM2 right   Tongue swollen and painful, throat obstructed, sores in mouth, excessive thirst, vomiting, diarrhoea.

HAI QUAN   SEA SPRING
XM3   Excessive thirst, throat obstructed, tongue swollen and painful, vomiting, diarrhoea.

Ear
ER JIAN   EAR POINT
XE1   Film over eyes.

Back
HUA TUO   FLOWERY HUMP
XB1   Coughing, dyspnoea, asthma, pain in back and loins, all mild complaints.
(These points are about half an inch on either side of the spines of the thoracic and lumbar vertebrae. A total of 34 points.)

PI GEN   OBSTRUCTION ROOT
XB2   Indigestion, feeling as if food does not pass through.

SI HUA   THE FOUR FLOWERS
XB3   Exhaustion, Qi weak, blood weak, bones weak, coughing phlegm, dyspnoea, emaciation.
(Another name for the two diaphragm and two gall bladder associated points: B17 and B19.)

Arm
SHI XUAN   TEN PROCLAMATIONS
XA1   Delirium, fainting, hysteria, epilepsy.
(Beneath the middle of the nail at the tips of the ten fingers.)

SI FENG   FOUR CRACKS

XA2   Pyloric stenosis ? throat, larynx.
(Middle of the palmar crease of the proximal-phalangeal joint. None for the thumb.)

ZHOU JIAN   ELBOW POINT

XA3   Adenitis.

Leg

HE DING   CRANE SUMMIT (BIRD)

XL1   Pain in knee, weakness of legs.

NEI XI YAN   INNER KNEE EYE

XL2   Pain and numbness in knee, difficulty in bending or flexing knee, knee swollen and painful.

LAN WEI   INTESTINE TAIL (APPENDIX)

XL3   Appendicitis.

NEI HUAI JIAN   INNER ANKLE POINT

XL4   Toothache in lower jaw, muscular cramp medial side of leg.

WAI HUAI JIAN   OUTER ANKLE POINT

XL5   Muscular cramp lateral side of leg, beri-beri.

A General Survey of Common Diseases and their Treatment by Acupuncture

(CHANGJIAN JIBING SHENJIU ZHILIAO BIANLAN)

COMPILED BY: THE PEKING SCHOOL OF CHINESE MEDICINE
PUBLISHED BY: THE PEOPLE'S HYGIENE PUBLISHING
HOUSE, PEKING, 1960

Acupuncture Points used in the Treatment of Specific Diseases or Symptoms

TAKEN FROM THE CASE HISTORIES OF DR. FELIX MANN
AND OTHER EUROPEAN DOCTORS
PRACTISING ACUPUNCTURE

Section 2 is envisaged as an extension to Section 1, mainly from the point of view of enlarging the variety of acupuncture points that may be used in a certain disease. For this reason only combinations of acupuncture points not mentioned in Section 1 have been included. The symptomatology of the individual point should determine which acupuncture point to use.

General Diseases

1. INFLUENZA, COLDS and related conditions   *GAN MAO*

Section 1

CAUSE OF DISEASE	SYMPTOMS	DIAGNOSTIC FEATURES	MAIN POINTS	SECONDARY POINTS
1. Affected by Wind Evil.	Dislikes the cold; fever; headache; clear mucus flows from nose; sneezing; nose blocked.	Pulse Floating; tongue slightly furred white.	Gv14 B12 T5 G20 Li4 B11	S8 Gv23 Li20
2. Affected by Wind and Cold.	Head and body painful; fever; dislikes cold.	Pulse Floating and Tight; tongue slightly furred white.	as above	Gv16 S36 XH3
3. Affected by Wind and Heat.	Headache; fever; mouth parched; eyes red.	Pulse Floating and Overflowing; tongue slightly furred yellow.	as above	Li11 XH3 (let blood)
4. Affected by Seasonal Evil.	Sudden high fever; head and nape of neck painful; body painful; breathing harsh; coughs up thick sputum; throat painful; eyes red; face flushed.	Pulse Floating and Overflowing; tongue furred yellow; chest melancholy.	as above	L7 L9 L11 L10 B13 Gv13
5. Affected by Wind and Damp	Headache; neck stiff; joints swollen and painful; no thirst.	Pulse Floating, Slow but Weak-floating; tongue white; no thirst; joints swollen and painful.	as above	Gv16 Li11 G34
6. Dormant Evil.	Headache; heart troubled; Shen weary; troubled sleep; urine red; mouth dry; no wish to drink; delirious speech.	Pulse Rapid; tongue red.	as above	Li11 B54
7. Summer-heat and Wind on exterior of body.	Headache; no sweating; heart distressed.	Pulse Floating but Weak-floating; tongue slightly red and yellow.	as above	Cx6

INFLUENZA
Cx6 Li4 L7
Li20
S16 G20
B11 B12 B13
The Yu points

SHIVERING
T5 K1 Cv12 B54 L10 Liv2 S36 Gv16 G25
Si14 S12 Sp9

2. PAROTITIS *ZHA SAI*

Section 1

CAUSE OF DISEASE	SYMPTOMS	DIAGNOSTIC FEATURES	MAIN POINTS	SECONDARY POINTS
Warm Poison erupts on jaws and neck.	Swelling from behind ears to nape of neck and from in front of ears to the jaw; body hot; spontaneous sweating.	Pulse Rapid; tongue red.	G20 Li4 L7	T17 T5

Section 2

MUMPS
T5 Li4 Si3

INSUFFICIENT SALIVA
Liv4

3. COUGH *KE SOU*

Section 1

CAUSE OF DISEASE	SYMPTOMS	DIAGNOSTIC FEATURES	MAIN POINTS	SECONDARY POINTS
1. Wind and Cold invade lungs.	Coughing; nose blocked; sneezing; dislikes cold; fever.	Pulse Floating; tongue slightly furred white.	G20 B12 B13	T5 L8
2. Wind and Heat injure lungs.	Coughing; mouth parched; body hot; sweating.	Both Inch Pulses Large; tongue furred white and slightly yellow.	B13 B12 Li4 L7	T5
3. Lung meridian Dry and hot.	Sputum difficult to cough up; sputum yellow; slight fever; palms of hands hot.	Right Inch Pulse Overflowing and Large; tongue furred yellow and white but dry.	B13 B12 Li4 L7	Cv22
4. Phlegm hot, obstructed and Full.	Coughing; chest melancholy; thick sputum causes obstruction and is difficult to cough up.	Pulse Slippery and Full; tongue yellow and greasy; stools hard; urine red.	Li4 L7 L5	S36 Sp9 T6

CAUSE OF DISEASE	SYMPTOMS	DIAGNOSTIC FEATURES	MAIN POINTS	SECONDARY POINTS
5. Cough due to Empty lung. (Note 1)	Continuous coughing; short of breath; Shen weary; movement causes dyspnoea; mouth parched; throat dry.	Pulse Empty.	B37 B38 Cv6	Cv12 S36
6. Cough due to Exhausted lung. (Note 2)	Continuous cough; blood in sputum; cheeks red; body emaciated; hot and flushed after midday.	Six Pulses Empty and Rapid; appearance haggard.	B37 B38 Gv12	S25 Cv6 S36

NOTES

1. *'Empty Lung: the Empty Lung is caused by a slight weakness in the lung Qi. Its symptoms are: light breathing, voice low and weak, skin dry and withered, frequent sweating, face dry and white, body fears the cold.'* (*Jianshi*)

2. *'Exhausted Lung: one of the Five Exhaustions (i.e. exhaustion of the Five Zang Organs: see Glossary). It is caused by damage to the Qi by Grief and Worry. The Symptoms are: gathering of the skin, loss of hair on body, appearance haggard, shivering and dislike of cold, coughing.'* (*Jianshi*)

Note that both Empty Lung and Exhausted Lung are diseases in themselves and have other symptoms apart from the coughing discussed here.

Section 2

LARYNGITIS
K7 K3
Cv23 Cv22 Cv18
G20 B10
B11 B12 B13

TRACHEITIS
Li4 L2
Gv12 G12 Cx3

COUGH
Yu points as indicated by the pulse
L8 L10 B13
K19 S41 Si2
B18 Liv8 H5 Cx8

COUGH—cont.
Gv12 Cv17 L11
S14 S15 S12 S36 Li10
K1 Sp14 L4
G21 K26 K27
Cv23 S19 K22 Cx2

COUGH WITH EXCESSIVE EXPECTORATION OR MUCUS THAT CANNOT BE EXPECTORATED
K2 B60 K5
T16 B13
Si1 H9
Cv12 S40 Cv17
B38 Sp9 Cx6
G10 Cv28

4. APHONIA   *BAO YIN*

Section 1

CAUSE OF DISEASE	SYMPTOMS	DIAGNOSTIC FEATURES	MAIN POINTS	SECONDARY POINTS
Cool Wind restrained outside the body; lung Qi does not circulate.	Sudden loss of speech.	Onset of disease sudden, not gradual	Gv16 Cv23 Li4	T5 Cx5

HYSTERICAL APHONIA
K1 Liv1 L11 Li10
Li13 B10 Cv23 T17 Si15
Gv15 G12 Li17
Li4 K4 H5

5. DYSPNOEA, Asthma, Pneumonia, Bronchitis and similar conditions (Note 1)   *CHUAN*

Section 1

CAUSE OF DISEASE	SYMPTOMS	DIAGNOSTIC FEATURES	MAIN POINTS	SECONDARY POINTS
1. Wind and Cold restrict lungs.	Fever; dislikes the cold; no sweating; coughing; sputum rattles in bronchi; dyspnoea.	Pulse Floating and Wiry; tongue furred white.	B13 B12 Li4 K7 L7 L10	T5 Cv12
2. Fire depressed in lungs.	Dyspnoea; body hot; sputum difficult to cough up; mouth dry; face red; disease at its worst after midday.	Inch Pulse Rapid; tongue thinly furred and slightly yellow.	B13 B15 L5 L9 L10	Cx6 Si4 L1
3. Phlegm obstructed.	Dyspnoea; sputum rattles; chest-diaphragm blocked and melancholy.	Pulse Large and Slippery; tongue furred yellow and greasy.	Cv22 L5 Cx6	Cv12 S40
4. Phlegm in bronchi attacks upwards.	Inability to sleep due to coughing and difficult breathing; thin saliva causes blockage.	Inch and Connecting Pulses Deep and Wiry; tongue furred white but not parched.	Cv12 Liv13 L5	Cx6 S36 B20
5. Qi rebels and attacks upwards.	Dyspnoea; no sputum; chest-ribs swollen and melancholy.	Inch Pulse Large; Foot Pulse Deep.	Cv17 B13 Gv10 S36	Cv22 L1
6. Lungs Empty and Qi weak.	Breathing short and difficult; unable to rest; night sweats; face white.	Pulse Empty; tongue substance pale.	B37 B38 Cv17 Cv6	S36 (moxa)
7. Kidney does not transmit Qi.	Qi does not return to its source; appearance haggard and emaciated; mouth dry; no wish to drink.	Both Foot Pulses have no source; tongue substance pale; urine clear and frequent.	B23 Cv4 K6	S36

CAUSE OF DISEASE	SYMPTOMS	DIAGNOSTIC FEATURES	MAIN POINTS	SECONDARY POINTS
8. Wind and Heat dyspnoea: Wind and Heat enter lungs.	Fever; dislikes the cold; face red; lips red; dyspnoea.	Tongue slightly furred white; Pulse Floating and Rapid.	Cv17 (moxa) B12 B13	Cv22 L7 S40
9. Wind and Cold dyspnoea: Wind and Cold injure lungs.	Dislikes the cold; dyspnoea; coughing; sputum watery; mouth not parched.	Pulse Floating and Slow; tongue furred white.	B12 B13 Cv6	Cv12 S36
10. Hot Interior dyspnoea: rich foods and intemperate eating lead to excess Heat inside body and cause dyspnoea.	Coughing; sputum glutinous; lips red; mouth parched; heart troubled; face red.	Pulse Slippery but does not show disease, which is indicated only by dyspnoea.	Cv12 Liv3	Cx6 S40
11. Empty dyspnoea: good constitution but Empty lungs; after prolonged illness may be prone to excessive colds and diarrhoea.	Breathing short and rapid; dyspnoea only intermittently; low-pitched voice; face white; Qi of spleen and stomach not connected.	Pulse Minute; tongue not furred.	B37 B38 Cv6	Li10
12. Phlegm-fluid dyspnoea: Phlegm-fluid remains in lungs (see Notes for No. 6 Gastritis).	Sputum rattles in throat; dyspnoea; unable to rest.	Pulse Slippery; tongue furred white and thick.	B13 Cv12 S40	Cv22
13. Chronic dyspnoea: Phlegm floating in lungs.	Unseasonal weather causes attacks which are intermittent and cease spontaneously; sputum rattles; dyspnoea; breathing difficult if attack is heavy; face white; lips colourless; all types of food may cause attack.	Pulse Wiry and Slippery or Wiry and Weak.	Cv22 B13 B38	S36 L5
14. Lung Qi does not accumulate.	Slight dyspnoea at all times but deteriorates with exertion; face white; breathing light; voice weak.	Pulse Minute and Weak.	Gv12 B13 B38	Cv6 S36
15. Horse-spleen Wind (Note 2): Cold Evil Visitor inside lungs; Cold changes to Heat.	Dyspnoea; chest withered; ribs on both sides collapse and become concave; Shen Qi melancholy and confused; appearance haggard and fierce.	Pulse Floating and Rapid.	Gv12 Cv17	T2 L10

CAUSE OF DISEASE	SYMPTOMS	DIAGNOSTIC FEATURES	MAIN POINTS	SECONDARY POINTS
16. Chronic dyspnoea brought on by external influences (e.g. other diseases).	Dyspnoea; sputum rattles; nose blocked; small amount of clear mucus from nose; nostrils sometimes red.	(no observations)	B38 (moxa) Gv16 B12 B13	S36 (moxa) T5 L7

NOTES

1. *The heading Chuan, normally means 'asthma' 'dyspnoea' 'difficult breathing' etc., though most commonly, 'asthma'. However, this sub-division clearly deals with pulmonary diseases other than asthma alone; consequently the Chinese word Chuan has been translated throughout as 'dyspnoea' to avoid giving the impression that we are here concerned with asthma alone.*

2. *'Horse-spleen Wind: popular name "severe dyspnoea" (Bao Chuan); symptoms: chest withered, breathing hurried, lungs swollen and full, ribs and nose agitated, Shen Qi (see Introduction) melancholy and distressed. Caused by Heat restrained in lungs.' (Jianshi)*

Section 2

ASTHMA
Often allergic—Liv8
Associated with fear, rigidity and gastric symptoms—K5
Anguish, a staring hollow look—L9
Local points—Cv17 K27 B11 Cv12 G25
Si14 B10 S36 G20
Cv17 H9 T3 L1
Cv13 L3
B51 Cv3 K1
Li8 Sp9 Gv10

BRONCHITIS
L7 Liv13 Li10 Li4
B11 B12 B13 B14 B36 B38
S12 Cv20
H3 Cv14

PNEUMONIA
L7 K3
Cv17
K24 K25 K26 K27 S16 S15 S14 S13

PNEUMONIA—cont.
B42 B43 B44 B36 B37
Li4 Li13
Sp21 Liv14 Sp17 Sp18

EMPHYSEMA
L11 Li1
L1 L2
Cv13 Cv16 Cv20 Cv21
K3 H3 L7
B17 B18 B22

PNEUMOCONIOSIS
K5 Cx6

PLEURISY
G37 G34 S40 Sp4
Liv3 Liv13
B43 Si9 Sp21 K23 S16
Li7 H3 Si4
B17 G35
S13 S15 S16
T5 K27 B11 B12 B13

6. GASTRITIS (Note 1) *TAN YIN*

Section 1

CAUSE OF DISEASE	SYMPTOMS	DIAGNOSTIC FEATURE	MAIN POINTS	SECONDARY POINTS
1. Phlegm-fluid: spleen loses its strength and movement.	Previously robust, now emaciated; chest-diaphragm swollen.	Pulse Wiry and Slippery.	B20 B21 Cv12 Liv13 S36	Cx6 L5
2. Suspended-fluid (Note 2): water stopped below ribs.	Ribs on both sides painful; water stops between ribs and is audible; excessive coughing and vomiting.	Pulse Deep and Wiry.	Liv13 Cv12 L5	S24 S28
3. Overflowing-fluid (Note 3): water and Damp leak into the four limbs.	Body painful and heavy; four limbs swollen and puffy.	Pulse Floating and Wiry.	B20 B23 Liv13 K7	T5 S36
4. Branch-fluid (Note 4): fluid stops between chest and diaphragm.	Coughing prevents rest; vomits mucus; body swollen and puffy.	Inch and Connecting Pulses Wiry and Full.	B17 Cv21 Liv13 Cv12	S28 Sp9

NOTES

1. *Gastritis is a somewhat fortuitous translation of the Chinese heading Tanyin, which literally means Phlegm-drink or Phlegm-fluid. No direct English equivalent exists. The Cihai gives: 'Chronic gastritis (normal Chinese medical term); fluid blocks the stomach and cannot be absorbed; it is audible. Ancient doctors called it Tanyin and it is also known as Tingyin (Stopped-fluid).' Under Tingyin is also given:*
'One of the symptoms of gastric inflammation or gastric catarrh. The function of the digestive juices is impaired so that fluid remains in the stomach. It also causes distress of the heart and vomiting of yellow or acid fluid. If acute, the noise of water can be heard when the body is shaken. Inflammation of the stomach must be cured before this complaint will cease.'
Under Tanyin, Jianshi gives:
'Thick and turbid fluids are called Tan, thin and clear fluids are called Yin; the two characters together are used as a short name for Tanyin Disease.'
Nos. 2, 3 and 4 are also given by Jianshi as variations of Tanyin, as below:
2. *Suspended-fluid: 'The Yang Qi of the Middle Warmer (see Glossary) is deficient, the blocked fluid cannot move to the bladder but is suspended beneath the ribs; this leads to coughing and vomiting and pain beneath the ribs.' (Jianshi)*
3. *Overflowing-fluid: The blocked fluid leaks into the skin of the limbs and cannot move down to the bladder as urine; it also cannot pass out of the body as sweat but remains in the body, causing swelling and pain.' (Jianshi)*
4. *Branch-fluid: 'One of the Tanyin Diseases, characterised by coughing, inability to sleep, dyspnoea, face and eyes swollen and puffy.*
Note also that Tanyin is given under item 12 of No. 5 Dyspnoea, as a cause of one of the pulmonary conditions listed there.

GLOBUS HYSTERICUS
L3 Cv14
Sp17 Cv12 H5

EPIGASTRIC PAIN
S45 Sp4 S25 Sp13
S36 K21 S21 L11
Cv12 Liv1

POOR DIGESTION
Liv13 Liv14
Sp15 S36 G25

POOR DIGESTION—cont.
B17

GASTRIC PTOSIS
Cv8 (S de Morant from Jap.)

ANOREXIA
S39 S45
Liv4
B17 B18 B19
Cv6

7. INTERMITTENT FEVERS, REMITTENT FEVERS, MALARIA and related conditions
NUE JI

Section 1

CAUSE OF DISEASE	SYMPTOMS	DIAGNOSTIC FEATURES	MAIN POINTS	SECONDARY POINTS
1. Affected by Wind and Cold.	Dislikes the cold; fever at regular intervals; desires to vomit; head dizzy.	Pulse Wiry; tongue furred white; side of tongue purple.	Gv14 Gv13 Cx5 T6 Si3	Gv16 Li4 Li11
2. Affected by Damp and Heat.	During attacks patient alternates rapidly between extremes of heat and cold; sweating relieves attack; great thirst; patient hot more than cold.	Left Pulse Wiry; tongue purple and slightly furred.	as above	Li4 Li11 S36
3. Attack caused if Dormant Qi exposed to Summer-heat.	Bones and joints painful; occasional vomiting; continually hot, never cold; muscles and flesh waste away.	Pulse normal; mouth parched; tongue furred yellow and greasy.	as above	B11 K6
4. Fever due to tiredness; Yin Qi ceases to function, only Yang Qi in operation.	Patient continually hot, never cold; mouth dry and hot.	Pulse Overflowing.	as above	XH2 Li4
5. Starvation or immoderate eating and drinking.	Patient feels hot and cold simultaneously; bouts of fever at regular intervals; stomach obstructed and full; dislikes food; breath putrid.	Pulse Wiry, Slippery and Full; tongue thickly furred and greasy.	as above	Cv12 S44 Sp4
6. Recurrent fever brought on by exhaustion; fever all day long; spleen and stomach Qi Empty.	Hot and cold simultaneously and at regular intervals; bout lasts whole day; limbs weary; fluctuation in temperature slight; sweating; dyspnoea.	Pulse Empty; tongue pale.	as above	B20 Liv13 L8 XB2

8. DYSENTERY   *LI JI*

Section 1

CAUSE OF DISEASE	SYMPTOMS	DIAGNOSTIC FEATURES	MAIN POINTS	SECONDARY POINTS
1. Cold dysentery: Zang organs Cold and Empty; this also causes cold in rest of body.	Face and lips blue-green and white; likes warm fluids; abdomen painful; intestinal noises; diarrhoea; if severe, feet and hands become cold; eyes prominent and red; stools like those of a duck.	Pulse Deep; tongue not furred.	S25 Cv6	B25 B29
2. Heat dysentery: Warmth congealed.	Fever; tongue red; lips burning; likes cold fluids; abdomen painful; incessant diarrhoea; small quantities of red urine; bowel painful and heavy.	Pulse Rapid; tongue thickly furred yellow.	Cv12 S25 Li4	Sp2 S44
3. Periodic dysentery: affected by Wind Evil from outside and injured by cold from within.	Fever; no sweating; whole body painful; diarrhoea and vomiting; abdomen painful; bowel heavy.	Pulse Floating and Slippery	B12 Cv12 T5	Li4 S36
4. Dysentery with trismus: Great Poison rushes into stomach; diarrhoea injures Yin.	Body hot; tongue red; lips red; diarrhoea without having eaten; likes cold fluids.	Pulse Rapid.	B20 B21 Cv12 S25	K7 Sp4
5. Nourishment dysentery: caused by food and water.	Diarrhoea; abdomen painful; bowel heavy.	Pulse Slowed-down.	B20 B21 Cv11	B25 B29
6. Chronic dysentery.	Intermittent dysentery may continue for 6–12 months; face yellowish-white; eats and drinks normally.	Pulse Fine and Rapid.	B20 B23 Cv4	K2 Sp4
7. Five-colour dysentery: due to use of purgative medicine or incomplete coagulation of food in bowel.	Stools of various colours, purulent and bloody.	Both Foot Pulses Fine.	B25 B27	S36 S25

97

DYSENTERY
Liv6 Sp6
Cv12 S36 S28 S39 K21 Cv6
T5 Cx6
S11 Gv1 K7
B62 Li4 G26 Liv2

9. DIARRHOEA *XIE XIE*

Section 1

CAUSE OF DISEASE	SYMPTOMS	DIAGNOSTIC FEATURES	MAIN POINTS	SECONDARY POINTS
1. Damp diarrhoea: cold produced by food and drink, sitting on damp surface, or excessive drinking of alcohol.	Limbs weary; stools watery; dysuria; insipid taste in mouth; inability to taste; chest-diaphragm suffering and melancholy; abdomen painful.	Pulse Weak-floating and Blocked; tongue furred, dirty and greasy.	Cv12 S25 B20 B25	Cv9 S36 Sp6
2. Fire diarrhoea: caused by overflowing of Heat, or by eating bitter, hot foods and excessive drinking of alcohol; Fire in body depressed and congealed.	Precipitous diarrhoea; abdomen painful; stools hot and foul-smelling; rectum burning and painful; burning pain in bowel during passing of stools; mouth parched; dreads the heat.	Tongue purple and furred yellow; small quantities of red urine; Pulse Deep and Rapid.	Cv12 S25 S36 S44	Li11 Li4 Sp9 S39
3. Food diarrhoea: excessive eating and drinking; food accumulates and congeals and is not broken down.	Belching; abdomen full; stools putrid and glutinous.	Pulse Full and Large; tongue furred, rough and yellow.	Cv13 Cv12 S25 Liv13	Cx6 S36 S37 S39
4. Water diarrhoea: food and water produce cold; water accumulates and is not digested.	Intestinal noises; lower abdomen painful; diarrhoea frequent and completely liquid; mouth parched despite drinking; dislikes cold.	Pulse Slow; tongue furred white and greasy.	Cv12 S25 B20 B23	Cv9 S28 S36 Sp6
5. Summer-heat diarrhoea: Summer-heat Qi damp, remains in intestines and stomach.	Face dirty; sweating; mouth parched; heart anxious; abdomen rumbles like thunder; stools watery.	Pulse Weak-floating; tongue furred and greasy.	Cv12 S25 B20 B25	Cx7 S36 Sp6

CAUSE OF DISEASE	SYMPTOMS	DIAGNOSTIC FEATURES	MAIN POINTS	SECONDARY POINTS
6. Phlegm diarrhoea: Damp and Phlegm flowing; large intestine not strong, allowing food to slip out as diarrhoea.	Intermittent diarrhoea; chest melancholy; food only slightly digested; patient may wish to vomit phlegm.	(no observations)	Cv12 S25 B25	Cx6 S36 S40
7. Cold diarrhoea: spleen Yang Empty and Cold.	Intestinal noises; severe pain in intestines; stools like those of a duck; dislikes the cold.	Pulse Slow; urine white.	Cv12 Cv6 Liv13 B20 B21	S25 B25 S36 Sp6
8. Spleen diarrhoea: spleen Empty; Pure Yang cannot ascend, thus producing diarrhoea.	Abdomen Empty and Full(?); diarrhoea after meals; patient appears emaciated; no strength; Jing Shen failing; stomach transmits Qi inadequately.	Pulse Empty and Pliable; no variations in colour of tongue (i.e. whole tongue of uniform colour).	Gv20 Cv12 Liv13 B21 B20	S25 Cv4 S36 Sp6
9. Kidney diarrhoea: kidney Empty and Cold; Yang Qi deficient.	Diarrhoea on rising in the morning (the so-called 'Fifth watch of the night diarrhoea'); limbs weary and cold; dislikes the cold; abdomen rumbles.	Pulse Empty and Weak; no variations in colour of tongue.	Cv12 Liv13 Cv8 B20 B23	Gv20 Cv4 S36 K6
10. Slippery diarrhoea: disease persists for long time; intestines slippery and weak.	No control of bowel action when passing stools.	Pulse Empty and Pliable; no variations in colour of tongue.	Gv20 Cv12 Cv6 B20 B23	B44 Gv4 Gv1 Cv8 S36

Section 2

COLITIS
K5 B23
Liv11 Liv2 Liv8
S25 S27 Cv12 Cv4
Sp9 K2 B65

COLITIS—cont.
L9 B54 Li11 S36
Sp1 Sp3 S44
Sp4 G41 Sp14 K14
K7 Cv9 B35

10. CHOLERA   *HUO LUAN*

Section 1

CAUSE OF DISEASE	SYMPTOMS	DIAGNOSTIC FEATURES	MAIN POINTS	SECONDARY POINTS
1. Affected by Wind and Cold from outside the body; inside the body food and	Vomiting; diarrhoea; vomitus like dirty water; dislikes the cold; fever; muscular spasms in severe cases.	Pulse Deep and Wiry; tongue furred white and slippery.	Cv12 S25 S36 S44	B57 Sp4

CAUSE OF DISEASE	SYMPTOMS	DIAGNOSTIC FEATURES	MAIN POINTS	SECONDARY POINTS
drink are obstructed; the Pure and Impure Qi contest; stomach and intestines are not in accord.			T5	
2. Affected by Summer-heat Evil.	Fever; no sweating; excessive vomiting; muscular spasms in severe cases; fingers cracked and shrivelled.	Pulse Floating and Wiry; tongue furred white.	XA1 S25 Li4 S36	B57 Cv12
3. Summer-heat attacks inside the body.	Mouth parched; heart troubled; body hot; sweating; vomiting; diarrhoea; limbs cold; spasms of limbs; eyes sunken.	Pulse Empty and Large or Weak-floating; face red; small quantities of urine.	L5 B54 (let blood) Li4 Cv12 S36	S44 S25 B57
4. Cold and Damp injure spleen.	Abdomen painful; vomiting; diarrhoea; hands and feet cold; muscular spasms in severe cases.	Pulse Deep and Fine; tongue furred greyish-white and not parched.	Cv8 Cv4 B20 B25	Cv6 S25 S36 B57

11. CHOLERA SICCA   *GAN HUO LUAN*

Section 1

CAUSE OF DISEASE	SYMPTOMS	DIAGNOSTIC FEATURES	MAIN POINTS	SECONDARY POINTS
1. Sudden attack of Cold and Damp; impurities in the body are obstructed and do not descend.	Abdomen extremely painful; heart troubled, agitated and melancholy; patient wishes to vomit and defaecate but cannot.	Pulse Deep and Wiry but Slow; Pulse Buried in severe cases; limbs cold; tongue furred, greasy and moist.	XA1 (let blood) Cv12 Cv6 Cv4 Cv8	Li4 S36
2. Summer-heat is impure and attacks within the body, preventing ascent or descent of Qi.	Lines of pain running through the abdomen; patient wishes to vomit and defaecate but cannot.	Pulse Deep and Slippery; Pulse Buried in severe cases; tongue red and furred yellow.	XA1 L5 B54 (let blood) Cv12 Cx6	S36 S44 Sp4

12. VOMITING   *OU TU*

Section 1

CAUSE OF DISEASE	SYMPTOMS	DIAGNOSTIC FEATURES	MAIN POINTS	SECONDARY POINTS
1. Stomach hot: savoury	Vomiting immediately after meals;	Pulse Overflowing and Large;	Cx6	Cv22

CAUSE OF DISEASE	SYMPTOMS	DIAGNOSTIC FEATURES	MAIN POINTS	SECONDARY POINTS
foods collect and become hot; stomach loses control and causes vomiting.	vomitus hot and foul-smelling; likes the cold and dislikes the heat; mouth parched and thirsty.	tongue furred yellow and parched.	Cv12 S36	S44 XM2 (let blood)
2. Spleen cold: spleen and stomach Empty and Cold; Yang Qi does not circulate; food not digested; Yin Qi turbid, does not descend.	Vomits large amounts of gastric secretions mixed with saliva, which is clear and cold; violent vomiting after food in morning; vomitus not hot or foul-smelling; no thirst; likes heat and dislikes cold; limbs cold.	Pulse Slowed-down and Fine; tongue furred white.	Cv12 Liv13 Cv17 B20 B21 B23	Cx6 Cv13 S36 Sp6
3. Qi obstructed: heart anxious; Qi uneasy and rebels upwards against the stomach.	Vomiting immediately after eating; chest and abdomen bloated and melancholy; obstruction below ribs; mouth bitter and hot; head and nape of neck may be painful, or not painful but swollen.	If hot: Pulse Wiry and Slippery; tongue furred yellow and burning.	Hot: Cx6 Cv12 S36	Hot: G34 Li4 Liv2 S41 XM2
	Patient may be either hot or cold: If hot: vomitus hot and foul-smelling; dislikes the heat; thirsty. If cold: vomits large amounts of clear fluid; no thirst; dislikes cold, likes heat.	If cold: Pulse Fine; tongue furred white.	Cold: Cx6 Cv12 S36 B17 Liv13 (moxa)	Cold: B18 B20 B21 Liv2 S44
4. Phlegm-fluid: (see Note to No. 6 Gastritis): previously body contained much Phlegm; spleen Yang may be immobile.	Vomiting if cold; vomits phlegm and saliva; no appetite; chest-diaphragm full and melancholy.	Pulse Slow and Slippery; tongue furred white.	Cx6 Cv12 S36 S40	Cv6 B17 B20 B21
5. Food accumulation: excessive eating causes accumulation and failure to digest.	Chest-diaphragm bloated and melancholy; dislikes smell of food; stools usually hot and foul-smelling; lines of pain in abdomen in more severe cases; vomitus putrid.	Pulse Full and Rough; tongue thickly furred and greasy.	Cx6 Cv12 Liv13 S36	Li4 Cv21 G34 Sp4
6. Middle Empty: spleen and stomach Empty and Weak; the Transforming Action of Qi is not effective (see Introduction).	Food cannot pass beyond the stomach which rebels and causes vomiting; limbs and body weary; body emaciated.	Pulse Empty and Fine; tongue thickly furred and greasy.	Cv12 Liv13 B20 B21	S25 S36 Sp6

AT CERTAIN TIMES AFTER S. DE MORANT
Acid vomiting at night—G23 G24
Vomiting with pyloric spasm—K21
Food vomited several hours after eating—G30
Vomiting after meals—Liv13
Vomiting, shoulder pain, food undigested—B22
Water brash—B13 Liv14 Liv2 Sp6

HAEMATEMESIS
B17 B18
Spl T5

13. HICCOUGH *E NI*

Section 1

CAUSE OF DISEASE	SYMPTOMS	DIAGNOSTIC FEATURES	MAIN POINTS	SECONDARY POINTS
1. Food produces cold; stomach may be Empty, and Cold.	Breath travels downwards then immediately upwards producing a short, sharp noise on leaving the mouth. Special symptoms: gullet swollen and full; hiccough may be cured by drinking hot water.	Pulse Slow and Fine; tongue thinly furred white.	B20 B21 Cv12	S25 S36
2. Liver Fire rises.	As above. Special symptoms: thirst.	Pulse Wiry and Rapid; tongue furred yellow.	B18 Liv2 Cx6	S36 G34
3. Spleen and stomach Qi Empty and weak.	As above. Special symptoms: noise slight; breathing light.	Pulse Minute or Fine.	B38 B17 Cv17 Cv6	S36
4. Stomach Hot, Dry and Full.	As above. Special symptoms: noise loud; breathing heavy; constipation.	Pulse Slippery and Full.	Cv12 S25 Cx6	L7 S36 S44

Section 2

HICCOUGH
B38
Cv12 Li9 K17
Liv13 Liv14 B17

HICCOUGH—cont.
Cx8 Li5 Cv17
Sp3 B19

14. NAUSEA AND VOMITING   *FAN WEI*

Section 1

CAUSE OF DISEASE	SYMPTOMS	DIAGNOSTIC FEATURES	MAIN POINTS	SECONDARY POINTS
1. Middle Warmer Empty and Cold.	Food rejected on entering stomach.	Pulse Slow and Weak; tongue pale.	Cv12 Liv13 B20 B21	S36 Sp6
2. Middle Warmer Cold and Empty; much Phlegm; Qi obstructed.	Vomits phlegm and saliva.	Pulse Weak; tongue furred and greasy.	G21 Cv17 Cv6 Cv12	Cx6 S36 S40
3. Stomach Empty; Qi obstructed.	Vomiting and hiccough; chest full.	Pulse Weak; tongue pale.	Cv12 B21 K16	Cx6 S36
4. Cold Phlegm Visitor in Upper Warmer.	Coughing and vomiting.	Pulse Slippery; tongue furred and greasy.	G21 Cv17 B17 Cv12	S36 Sp4
5. Lower Warmer Empty and Cold; Fire weak; Earth sinking.	Food eaten in morning vomited in in evening.	Pulse Slow and Weak; tongue pale.	Cv6 Cv4 B20 B23	S36 Sp6
6. Spleen and stomach Qi Empty; True Yin dried up.	Chronic nausea; constipation.	Pulse Rough.	Cv12 Liv13	S36
7. Alcohol injures spleen.	Vomiting.	Pulse Slow and Weak; tongue furred white and greasy.	Cv12 Liv13 B20	Cx6 S36
8. Damp depressed, becomes Heat; stomach Fire rushes upwards.	Vomiting immediately after eating.	Pulse Rapid; tongue purple.	G21 Cv12 Liv13	Cx6 S36 S44

Section 2

NAUSEA, VOMITING	AEROGASTRIA	OESOPHAGEAL SPASM
Liv8 Liv14	L8 L10 Cx6	B38 Cv17
B62 Gv12	Liv14 G25 Liv13 Sp16	Sp6 B17
Cx6, S36	Cv12 Gv6 Cv12	K21 B45 Cx8
B17	Sp2 Sp4	G20 B18 Cv22 Li11 Sp5
Cx5 Li11 Sp5		
Si3 L7 Li4		
Cx8 Si1		
L9 Cx7		

15. GASTRALGIA *WEI TONG*

Section 1

CAUSE OF DISEASE	SYMPTOMS	DIAGNOSTIC FEATURES	MAIN POINTS	SECONDARY POINTS
1. Affected by Cold Evil from outside and by cold matter from within; Cold Visitor in stomach.	Stomach suddenly painful.	Pulse Deep and Tight.	Cv13 Cv12 Cv10 Cx6 S36 S25 Cv6	S34 S21
2. Stomach depressed and Hot.	Pain in stomach; feels extremely hot.	Pulse Slippery and Rapid; thirsty; tongue red; likes cool drinks.	as above	S44
3. Qi obstructed.	Stomach painful, swollen, full and uncomfortable.	Pulse Deep and Rough.	as above	B18 Liv13
4. Dead blood.	Pain in stomach at particular points which feel as though being pierced.	Pulse Rough; tongue black.	as above	B20 B21 B18 B19 B17
5. Stomach Empty.	Continuous pain in stomach; likes to press stomach to relieve pain.	Pulse Empty, Slowed-down and without strength; face white; small appetite.	as above	B20 B21 B18
6. Stomach Full and obstructed.	Stomach painful, obstructed and swollen; constipated.	Pulse Deep and Full; right Connecting Pulse has strength; tongue thickly furred yellow.	as above	S44

Section 2

PEPTIC ULCER

Acid-base imbalance: the kidneys and to some extent the lungs, keep the pH of the blood normal — K5 L9

Purely gastric type — S45

Really a hepatic disturbance, but has nearly indistinguishable symptoms — Liv8 G40
Abdominal type — Cx6 Cv12 Cv13 Cv10 S25 S36

A large proportion of patients with peptic ulcer respond to one of the above four combinations. There are of course in addition an infinite number of different combinations or variations:

B17 B18 B19 B20 B21 B22
B41 B42 B43 B44 B45
Gv6 Gv7 Gv8 Gv9

Any point on the upper abdomen may be used, according to its symptomatology. If the abdominal point is excessively tender or large, it should not be used, as it might easily cause an aggravation.

16. ABDOMINAL PAIN *FU TONG*

Section 1

CAUSE OF DISEASE	SYMPTOMS	DIAGNOSTIC FEATURES	MAIN POINTS	SECONDARY POINTS
1. Affected by Cold.	Lines of pain in abdomen; stools may be loose.	Pulse Deep and Slow; tongue furred white; likes heat and not thirsty.	Sp4 Cx6 S36 Cv12 Cv4 S25	
2. Qi of the Seven Emotions depressed.	Abdomen painful, obstructed and swollen; no appetite or thirst.	Pulse Deep; face haggard.	as above	
3. Empty and Cold.	Pain not severe.	Pulse Deep and Wiry; tongue pale; no thirst; urine clear; likes warmth; presses abdomen to relieve pain.	as above	
4. Food stopped up.	Abdomen painful, swollen and full; dislikes food; halitosis; saliva sour.	Pulse Deep and Slippery; tongue thickly furred and greasy; presses abdomen.	as above	S44
5. Inside Hot; Fire depressed.	Abdomen painful; vomiting; thirsty and likes cold drinks.	Pulse Rapid; tongue red; small quantities of red urine.	as above	Li4

Section 2

'TUMMY ACHE'
Sp4 Liv4
S37 Cv9 S22
B57 Cx6 Li8
S25 Sp6 Cv12 Liv13

ABDOMINAL DISTENSION
L9 Li11
Cv3 Cv5 Cv10 Cv12
Liv13

AEROCOLON
K8 S19 S29 Sp6
S36 Cv8 Li3 Liv3

17. INTESTINAL INFLAMMATION *CHANG YONG*

Section 1

CAUSE OF DISEASE	SYMPTOMS	DIAGNOSTIC FEATURES	MAIN POINTS	SECONDARY POINTS
Damp and Hot Qi obstructed and congealed.	Abdomen extremely painful when pressed; bowel action heavy.	Pulse Slow or Tight.	XL3	Li11 S36

Section 2

INTESTINAL SPASM
B62 Li4

18. CONSTIPATION *BIAN MI*

Section 1

CAUSE OF DISEASE	SYMPTOMS	DIAGNOSTIC FEATURES	MAIN POINTS	SECONDARY POINTS
1. Hot and Dry Yang congealed.	Faeces in bowels dry and congealed, and not passed.	Pulse Deep and Rapid and has strength; tongue furred yellow; abdomen swollen, obstructed and full.	T6 S25 B25 G34	Cv12 S36 Li4 S44
2. Cold and Dry Yin congealed.	Stools dense and congealed.	Pulse Deep and Slow and has strength; tongue thickly furred white; no appetite.	Cv12 Cv4 S25 B25	T6 S36 Sp6
3. Qi dense.	Qi penetrates and obstructs the frame of the body; stools dense and congealed.	Pulse Deep; chest-diaphragm obstructed and full; abdomen swollen.	Cv12 Cv6 T6 G34	Cx6 S36 Gv1 Liv1 S44
4. Blood dense.	Stools dense and congealed.	Pulse Empty and Large; tongue substance purple; mouth dry; heart troubled; sleep restless.	B17 B18 B15 T6	Cx7 Sp6
5. Wind dense.	Stools dense and congealed.	Pulse Floating and Wiry.	B12 B14 B25	T6 G34 S36 K3

Section 2

CONSTIPATION
Yin — T6 S36
Yang — Gv1 Liv1 G34
  (A. Chamfrault)
Weak abdominal muscles — Sp13
Distended abdomen — B28
Habitual constipation — T7 G34
K17 K16 B46 (S. de Morant).

CONSTIPATION—Cont.
Unable to pass motion — Sp6 B57 Cv6 B31
  (S. de Morant)
Liv13 Liv3 Sp3 Cv12
B57 K6
B23 B24 K15 K16

19. JAUNDICE *HUANG DAN*

Section 1

CAUSE OF DISEASE	SYMPTOMS	DIAGNOSTIC FEATURES	MAIN POINTS	SECONDARY POINTS
1. Damp and Heat jaundice: spleen and stomach Damp and Hot.	Eyes and body yellow; urine yellow; abdomen full; constipation.	Pulse Deep, Slippery and Full; tongue furred yellow and greasy.	Cv12 S36 Gv9 B19	Gv14 G34 S44 Sp4

CAUSE OF DISEASE	SYMPTOMS	DIAGNOSTIC FEATURES	MAIN POINTS	SECONDARY POINTS
2. Damp and Heat depressed inside the body; bladder Qi does not Transform.	Body and face completely yellow; dysuria.	(no observations)	B19 Gv9 B27 B28 Cv3	Cv12 S36 S28 Sp9
3. Yin yellow: spleen and kidney Empty and Cold; Damp is stored up and is not transformed.	Body and face yellow and of dark complexion; arms and legs cold from extremities to elbows and knees.	Pulse Deep and Fine; tongue pale and furred white; intestines melancholy; no appetite; no constipation.	Cv12 Gv9 B20 B23	Si4 S36 Sp9 Sp6
4. Nourishment jaundice: Damp, Heat and stale foods attack each other.	Stomach bitter and melancholy; head dizzy after eating; body and face hot.	Pulse Slippery; tongue furred, slippery and greasy.	Cv12 B19 B20 B21	Cx6 S36 L7 Li4 S44
5. Alcohol jaundice: excess of alcohol; Damp and Heat steaming	Heart melancholy and disordered; sometimes painful and hot and unable to eat, or having eaten wishes to vomit; soles of feet hot; dysuria; body and face yellow.	Pulse Wiry and Slippery; tongue furred, slippery and greasy.	Sp4 B19 Gv9 B54	Si4 B27 B28 Cv12 S36 Sp9
6. Woman-weary jaundice (Note 1): Heat Evil injures kidney.	Body yellow; forehead black; lower abdomen full; soles of feet hot; stools black and loose.	Pulse Deep, Fine and Rapid; tongue furred black and insipid.	B23 B67 Sp4	K6 K2

NOTES

1. *Mathews gives 'Woman-weary jaundice' as 'chlorosis' while Jianshi says simply 'a type of jaundice'. Although from the symptoms given here it seems unlikely that 'chlorosis' is correct, it is interesting to note that the modern Chinese term for that condition is 'withering yellow disease' whereas in English it is known as 'green sickness', (chlorosis).*

Section 2

JAUNDICE
Liv8 K5
G21 Si14
B44 S44 Li4 Cv12
Cx7 K7 Liv4

JAUNDICE—Cont.
Li2 Li13
Si8 G38 G40 Sp5 Liv8 B38 Sp10 B54
  (S. de Morant)

20. SWELLING OF ABDOMEN ONLY (Note 1)   *DAN FU TONG*

Section 1

CAUSE OF DISEASE	SYMPTOMS	DIAGNOSTIC FEATURES	MAIN POINTS	SECONDARY POINTS
1. Abdomen swelling: the Swelling Disease has its roots in the spleen where the Yin is injured. Although the stomach transmits Nourishment, the spleen does not transform it (i.e. into Qi, Blood, Ying, Wei etc. see Introduction); Anger may injure the liver and gradually encroach upon the spleen, the spleen is extremely Empty so Yin and Yang do not meet; Pure and Impure Qi are mixed together, so the Way cannot be penetrated, and this causes Heat; Damp and Heat are both generated, so the abdomen becomes swollen.	Abdomen swollen and Empty; skin taut; if the patient eats in the morning he cannot do so in the evening. (If the navel protrudes (Note 2) dark veins appear on the abdomen and the skin is like oil, then the disease is severe and cannot be cured).	Pulse Floating and Large in mild cases, Empty and Small in severe cases.	Cv12 B20 B23 B22 Liv13 Cv9 Cv6	Cx6 K7 Sp4 S36 Sp6
2. Qi depressed: great anger or frustration cause liver Fire to move vigorously and make the sides of the body painful. Dead blood: bad blood remains below the ribs and makes the sides of the body painful; extreme pain when pressed.	Either right or left or both sides of body painful.	Qi painful; pain intermittent; abdomen swollen; slight relief from pain if warm; pain circulates; Inch Pulse Wiry. Blood painful: painful whether pressed or not; pain continuous; no swelling; dead blood causes obstruction; disease mild during day, severe at night; fever after midday; Pulse Short and Rough.	Cv12 Cv6 B18 Liv13 B17 B18 Liv13	Liv14 Sp4 Cx6 S36 Liv14 B54 G40 Cx6
3. Swelling in abdomen only: violent anger injures liver; anxiety injures spleen. (This	Only abdomen, not limbs, swollen. The Yi Zhi (Purpose of Healing) says: 'There is a disease called 'Spider poison swelling' in which	Abdomen visibly swollen: ribs on both sides must be examined in order to make sure there is no swelling and	Cv12 Cv6 Liv13 B20	S36 Sp6 Sp9

CAUSE OF DISEASE	SYMPTOMS	DIAGNOSTIC FEATURES	MAIN POINTS	SECONDARY POINTS
disease is popularly called the 'spider drum' disease.)	only the abdomen is swollen and the four limbs are very emaciated.'	pain; and the abdomen should be examined to make sure there is no accumulation of fluid. The ribs should also be examined for symptoms of other diseases which may be caused by the liver and spleen.	B18 B22 Cv9	

NOTES

1. *In this case the English title is a direct translation of the Chinese. The condition should be contrasted with Nos. 21 and 22.*

2. *The 'protruding navel' is also found as a condition in itself, occurring in children. The protrusion may apparently vary greatly in size. In fact the same term, Qi Tu Chu, is now used for 'umbilical hernia': in this case the modern and the traditional use of a Chinese term are virtually identical, but this is uncommon. The older usage is rarely as precise as the modern one, and not infrequently has a completely different meaning.*

Section 2

ASCITES
Cv9 S28 Sp6 G28
K7

21. QI-ACCUMULATION DISEASES (Mainly gastric) (Note 1)   *JI JU*

Section 1

CAUSE OF DISEASE	SYMPTOMS	DIAGNOSTIC FEATURES	MAIN POINTS	SECONDARY POINTS
1. Immoderate eating and drinking gradually cause blockage and accumulation of Qi.	Hard obstruction in abdomen which is swollen, painful and melancholy.	Pulse Rough; tongue thickly furred.	Cv12 Liv13 XB2 B20 B21	S36 Sp4
2. Phlegm-fluid, blood and Qi accumulated.	Chest and abdomen obstructed.	Pulse Deep, Full and Fine.	Cv12 Liv13 B20 B18 XB2	Cx6 S36 S40 S44
3. The Five Exhaustions and the Seven Injuries; dried blood within the body.	Body emaciated; abdomen full; cannot eat and drink; skin dry and scaly; both eyes black.	Pulse Rough.	Cv12 Liv13 B17 B18 XB2	Sp10 K6 B54 S36 Sp6

CAUSE OF DISEASE	SYMPTOMS	DIAGNOSTIC FEATURES	MAIN POINTS	SECONDARY POINTS
4. Affected by the Seven Emotions.	Acute dyspnoea; chest-diaphragm listless; heart distressed; no appetite.	Pulse Rough; no indication of accumulated Qi; Qi sometimes scattered, sometimes accumulated.	Cv13 Liv13 Cv6 B13 B17	Cx6 S36 S44
5. Qi Cold and accumulated.	Limbs obstructed; bowel cold and constipated.	Pulse Rough.	Cv12 Cv6 S25 B25	S36 Sp6
6. Spleen weak and loses its movement; Empty Evil becomes accumulated.	Obstruction in bowel; emaciated, weak and weary.	Pulse Fine and Rough.	Cv12 Liv13 B20 B21 B23 XB2	S36 S40 Sp4
7. A prolonged accumulation causes Gan (see No. 90 GAN JI) and activates the liver Fire.	Cheeks swollen; mouth wasted away; teeth and gums rotten; constipated.	Pulse Wiry and Rapid; mouth hot, thirsty and painful.	Cv12 Liv13 S25 B20 B19 B22	Li4 S36 G34 Liv2

NOTES

1. *Separately Ji, and Ju, have a more precise meaning than is evident here. According to Jianshi: 'An accumulation of Qi is called Ji; it occurs in a definite place and its pain is not far from that place. A gathering together of Qi is called Ju; it does not occur in any definite place and its pain has no fixed location. The combination of Ji and Ju means that a Qi disease of accumulating, obstructing, gathering and congealing affects the Zang and Fu organs.'*

22. OEDEMA *SHUI ZHONG*

Section 1

CAUSE OF DISEASE	SYMPTOMS	DIAGNOSTIC FEATURES	MAIN POINTS	SECONDARY POINTS
Fluid causes obstruction inside the body; Wind and Cold restrained outside the	Eyes, limbs, abdomen and genitals all swollen; if the disease attacks upwards it causes difficult breathing, coughing and vomiting; if it	1. Empty Swelling: disease usually protracted; fatigue; appearance dejected; voice weak and hesitant; Pulse	B13 B23 B20 B28	Cv6 Cv4 Cv3 S36

CAUSE OF DISEASE	SYMPTOMS	DIAGNOSTIC FEATURES	MAIN POINTS	SECONDARY POINTS
body; the Triple Warmer transforms but does not activate; the skin becomes swollen.	collects below, retention of urine occurs.	Empty. 1a. Lung Qi Empty and unable to circulate; region below the heart rebellious and full; Qi attacks chest. 1b. Spleen Qi Empty and unable to vaporize; water saturates the middle of the body. 1c. Kidney Qi Empty and unable to activate the water; oliguria.	Cv9 S28 Cv8	Sp6 Sp9 K7
		2. Full Swelling: usually severe; Pulse always Abundant; oliguria and constipation.	Li4 L7 Sp9 K7 S28 Cv9	S43 S36 Sp6 B27 Gv26

Section 2

OEDEMA OF FEET
G31 Sp4 Sp9 G30
B54 B57 B58 B62

CARDIAC OEDEMA
H7 B15 B23
H9 K8
S36 S43 G30 Li4

CARDIAC OEDEMA—cont.
Sp6 T7 Cv5

VARICOSE VEINS
Only slight effect
Gv14 Gv12 G21 Gv4
Plus local points on legs (A. Chamfrault)

23. PENETRATING WIND (Cerebral Haemorrhage: see Note 1.)   *ZHONG FENG*

Section 1

CAUSE OF DISEASE	SYMPTOMS	DIAGNOSTIC FEATURES	MAIN POINTS	SECONDARY POINTS
1. Penetrating the Luo: Wind Evil penetrates the Luo.	Mouth and eyes awry; flesh and skin numb; movement causes pain.	Pulse Floating, Wiry and Anxious.	S6 S4 T17 Li4 L7 S36	Gv26 Cv24 G14 S2 G20 Si18 S42 Li20
2. Penetrating the meridians: Wind	Hands and feet paralysed; tongue feeble.	Pulse Deep and Wiry.	Gv20 Gv16	G20 T5

CAUSE OF DISEASE	SYMPTOMS	DIAGNOSTIC FEATURES	MAIN POINTS	SECONDARY POINTS
penetrates the meridians.			Li15 Li11 Li4 G30 G34 G39	Si3 G21 Li10 S36 G31 B60
3. Penetrating the Zang and Fu organs.	Patient suddenly collapses and becomes unconscious; mouth tightly closed and unable to open; face red; hands tightly clenched; breathing harsh.	Pulse Slippery and Un-yielding.	all or any of Category 1 points. XA1 (let blood) Gv20 Gv26	Li4 S6 K1
4. (no observations)	Special symptoms: eyes and mouth wide open; no control of body; urinary incontinence; heavy sweating.	Pulse Minute and Weak.	Cv8 Cv6 Cv4	Gv26 Cx9 Gv20

NOTES

1. *Although this subdivision seems in fact to be concerned with various results of cerebral haemorrhage, in order to make use of the material supplied here, it is more profitable to retain the Chinese terminology and seek to understand the traditional Chinese interpretation of the cause of the symptoms listed. It is unlikely that the Chinese knew of the existence of cerebral haemorrhage until fairly recent times, but this in no way effects the validity of the argument: cerebral haemorrhage, or any other 'cause' of this condition, would simply be regarded as a result of the primary cause, in this case Wind Evil.*

Moreover 'cerebral haemorrhage' does not cover all that is implied in the term Penetrating Wind; for instance the Cihai says:

'Chinese medicine says the cause of the disease is Wind (see Introduction); Western medicine says it is caused by cerebral haemorrhage. There are also conditions (embraced by the term Penetrating Wind) due to bleeding in the stomach and intestines, and in the pericardium.'

24. SECONDARY PENETRATING WIND (Note 1) *LEI ZHONG FENG*

Section 1

CAUSE OF DISEASE	SYMPTOMS	DIAGNOSTIC FEATURES	MAIN POINTS	SECONDARY POINTS
1. Fire penetrating: the Fire of the Five Desires erupts inside the body.	Sudden collapse and loss of con-sciousness; body hot; constipation.	Face red; tongue red; Pulse Overflowing and Rapid.	XA1 (let blood) Gv26 Gv20	Li4 K1 Cx9

CAUSE OF DISEASE	SYMPTOMS	DIAGNOSTIC FEATURES	MAIN POINTS	SECONDARY POINTS
2. Cold penetrating: Yin Cold penetrates the Zang organs.	Sudden lockjaw; hands and feet trembling; face sad and colourless.	Pulse Deep and Slow or Buried.	Cv4 Cv6 Cv12	Li4 Liv3 Gv26 Gv20
3. Food penetrating: excessive eating or drinking.	After eating patient suddenly becomes delirious; cannot speak; cannot raise limbs; chest and abdomen hard and full.	Pulse Deep and Full or Buried.	XA1 (let blood) Li4 Gv20 Gv26	Cx6 Cv12 S36
4. Emptiness penetrating: Qi Empty and extremely weary.	Sudden collapse and delirium; face pale and yellow.	Pulse Empty; tongue pale.	Cv6 Cv4 Cv12 Cv8	S36 Cx6
5. Qi penetrating: Qi of the Seven Emotions rebels.	Sudden delirium; Tide of Phlegm confined and obstructed; teeth tightly clenched; body cold.	Inch Pulse Deep.	Gv26 Gv20 XA1 Li4	S6 Cv22 S40
6. Summer-heat penetrating: Summer-heat Evil invades the interior of the body.	Shen Jing confused; severe sweating; dyspnoea; thirst.	Face dirty or red; Pulse Hollow and without strength.	XA1 Gv26 Li4	B54 (let blood) L5 S36

NOTES

1. *The term 'secondary' is a purely arbitrary one to make a distinction with No. 23 Penetrating Wind; the Chinese word Lei means something like 'in the same category as', 'similar to'. In fact the physiological causes of the symptoms of Secondary Penetrating Wind may have no connection whatsoever with cerebral haemorrhage (see Notes to No. 23); but to the Chinese mind are intimately bound up with Penetrating Wind. Jianshi says: 'This disease is similar to Penetrating Wind, but does not have the symptoms of hemiplegia and contortion of the eyes and mouth.'*

25. TRISMUS *KOU JIN*
Section 1

CAUSE OF DISEASE	SYMPTOMS	DIAGNOSTIC FEATURES	MAIN POINTS	SECONDARY POINTS
1. Wind and Cold stopped outside the body.	Teeth tightly clenched.	Unable to open mouth.	S6 Li4	T17 T5
2. Heat blazing and convulsed.	As above.	Unable to open mouth; mouth may be twisted.	S6 S7 T17	Li1 (let blood) T1 S36

FACIAL SPASM
L7 S40 T5
S6 Li4
Li20 S5

26. CONVULSIONS (allied to Insanity) (see Note 1) *DIAN, KUANG, XIAN*

Section 1

CAUSE OF DISEASE	SYMPTOMS	DIAGNOSTIC FEATURES	MAIN POINTS	SECONDARY POINTS
Dian: (Note 2) Principal causes: Heart Qi Empty; Phlegm Hot and abundant. Secondary causes: Fright; Anger; Qi and blood deficient; Phlegm remains surrounding the Luo; Excessive worry; Heart meridian stores Heat; Yin Empty; Shen Empty.	At first unhappy; head heavy and painful; eyes red; weeping; Shen foolish; speech incoherent; severe loss of balance and patient collapses; muscular spasms and rigidity.	Heavy Yin Dian: (Note 3) 1. Bone Dian: teeth and jaws diseases; space between skin and flesh full (Note 4); sweating; depression. 2. Sinew Dian: severe muscular spasms. 3. Blood-vessel Dian: severe loss of balance; blood-vessels in limbs swollen and full; patient may vomit phlegm. In cases where Qi descends and leaks away the disease is incurable. Pulse Large and Slippery, eventually returning to normal; in this case there is Qi in the stomach. If Pulse Small, Strong and Anxious, there is no cure and patient dies; in this case there is no Qi in stomach.	Gv12 Gv26 Cv12 H7	Cx6 Si3 S40
Kuang: (Note 5) Principal causes: Heat Evil in heart; Phlegm accumulates in the holes of the heart. Secondary causes: Upper Warmer Full; Large intestine and stomach meridians hot; Heat enters the Chong Mo; Fire excessive, mad and reckless;	Forgetful; prone to rage and fear; sleeps little; no appetite; previously a reputable person capable of rational thought and possessing knowledge and sound moral values; prone to use abusive language; does not rest day or night; fond of singing and music; moves about wildly and without pause; eats much; prone to see ghosts.	Wild speech; does not avoid vulgarity; if case is severe may remove clothes and walk about naked; may also climb to high places and sing.	Gv16 B15 Gv26 Cv12	Cx5 S40 Sp6

CAUSE OF DISEASE	SYMPTOMS	DIAGNOSTIC FEATURES	MAIN POINTS	SECONDARY POINTS
Frightened, sorrowful Phlegm accumulates; Animal Soul lost; Sorrow and pity move in the middle of the body and injure the Spiritual Soul. Excessive pleasure injures the Animal Soul.				
Xian: (Note 6) Principal causes: kidney meridian ceases to function; the two Yin are agitated and become Xian and Cold. The kidney Dragon Fire ascends and the liver Lightening follows in order to assist. Although all the forms of Xian have their origin in the kidney, their manifestations are according to the Five Zang: 1. Horse Xian (heart) 2. Ox Xian (spleen) 3. Pig Xian (kidney) 4. Chicken Xian (liver) 5. Sheep Xian (lung)	Spits saliva; Shen confused; suddenly does not know or recognise anything; trismus; convulsions lasting any length of time; after attacks behaves normally. 1. Patient opens mouth wide and shakes head; neighs like a horse; this corresponds to the heart. 2. Stares straight ahead; abdomen swollen; makes noise like an ox; corresponds to spleen. 3. Spits saliva; grunts like a pig; corresponds to kidney. 4. Shakes head to and fro; clucks like chicken; corresponds to liver. 5. Raises eyes and ejects tongue; bleats like a sheep; corresponds to lung.	**Yang Xian:** Phlegm hot, lodges in heart and stomach. Attack occurs when startled. Yin Xian also basically due to hot Phlegm. If doctor uses too much medicine (i.e. herbs, drugs, etc.) the spleen and stomach become Yin. When attack occurs in early morning, disease is in liver. When attack occurs in early evening, disease is in spleen. When attack occurs at dawn, disease is in gall-bladder. When attack occurs in middle of day, disease is in bladder. When attack occurs in late evening, disease is in stomach. When attack occurs in middle of night, disease is in kidney.	G20 Gv14 B15 H7	Cx5 Si3 S40 Liv2

NOTES

1. *As in the previous two diseases, we are here chiefly concerned with conditions of the brain. There are no exact equivalents for Dian, Kuang and Xian in European languages. From the symptoms it seems clear that both symptomatic and idiopathic fits are included — Blood-vessel Dian might possibly be hypertensive encephalopathy, whereas Xian seems more likely to be epilepsy. To the Chinese this is of no consequence, since primarily their classification of diseases is according to observed symptoms rather than etiology as recognised in the West.*

2. *Dian is defined as 'a type of nervous condition' by the Cihai. Note however that a modern Chinese medical word compounded of Dian and Xian is the normal term for epilepsy.*

3. *Heavy Yin Dian: i.e. Dian occurring in a person with an excess of Yin.*

4. *The 'space between the skin and flesh' is a common Chinese 'anatomical' term. (See Introduction under Wei.)*

5. *Kuang is the common Chinese word for 'mad' 'insane' in a general sense. More precise terms such as schizophrenia, paranoia etc. may well be included in Kuang, but are probably of less use here than the more vague 'insanity' — though conversely 'insanity' in English may embrace more than Kuang.*

6. *Xian is vaguely defined as 'fits' 'convulsions' 'epilepsy' etc.*

Section 2

MENTAL DISEASES
Depression — treat liver and gall bladder
Fears — treat kidney and bladder
Obsessions — treat spleen and stomach
Anguish — treat lung and large intestine
Emotional states — treat heart and small intestine
See pages 106–107 in my other book.

27. ZANG ORGANS AGITATED *ZANG ZAO*

Section 1

CAUSE OF DISEASE	SYMPTOMS	DIAGNOSTIC FEATURES	MAIN POINTS	SECONDARY POINTS
1. Liver Qi depressed and congealed; Ying and blood deficient.	Patient prone to grief and weeping; often stretches the body (as when tired).	Pulse Wiry; tongue red and not furred.	Gv26 H7 Gv20 Cv12 Cx7 K1 Gv14 B15	Li4 Liv3 Si3 S40

Section 2

EXCESSIVE NERVOUS TENSION
Si3 B62
Yu points.

28. INSOMNIA *SHI MIAN*

Section 1

CAUSE OF DISEASE	SYMPTOMS	DIAGNOSTIC FEATURES	MAIN POINTS	SECONDARY POINTS
1. Mental anxiety and weariness injure heart and spleen.	Patient startled and agitated; night-sweats; cannot sleep having woken; tired and lethargic; eats little; forgetful.	Pulse Weak; tongue pale.	H7 Sp6 B15 B20	H6 Si3 Cv4 S36
2. Heart blood deficient; Fluid dried up.	Shen Zhi ill at ease; palpitations of the heart; forgetful; constipated; sores in mouth and on tongue.	Pulse Fine and Rapid; tongue deep red; urine red; mouth dry.	B15 B23 H7 B42	Li4 S36 Sp6

116

CAUSE OF DISEASE	SYMPTOMS	DIAGNOSTIC FEATURES	MAIN POINTS	SECONDARY POINTS
3. Kidney water deficient; heart Fire burning.	Heart troubled; cannot sleep.	Pulse Rapid; tongue deep red.	B15 B23 Cx7 Sp6	H7 K6 S36
4. Weariness injures lungs; extreme weariness damages liver.	Empty exhaustion, Empty irritation (Note 1); cannot sleep.	Pulse Rapid; tongue deep red; slight fever.	H7 L9 Sp6 B13 B18	Cx6 S36 K6
5. Fright and fear.	Restless sleep; patient jumps up in alarm during dreams.	Pulse Wiry and Fine or Empty and Floating.	H7 L9 Sp6 B13 B19 B23	Li4 Liv3 B39 B42
6. Damp and Phlegm obstructed.	Cannot sleep peacefully at night; vomitus foul; Qi melancholy; chest-diaphragm not in order.	Pulse Slippery; tongue greasy; mouth acrid.	Cv12 B17 B20	Cx6 S36 S40 Sp6
7. Stomach not in harmony and has accumulation of food	Restless sleep; stomach swollen, melancholy and painful.	Pulse Full; tongue thickly furred.	Cv12 B20 B21 Cx6 S36	H7 Sp6 Sp1 S45

NOTES

1. 'Empty exhaustion, Empty irritation': as usual what is here a symptom is given by Jianshi also as a 'disease' in itself.
'Empty exhaustion' (Xu Lao) is an Exhaustion Disease (see Glossary) characterised by an Emptiness in the Qi, Blood, Fluid and Marrow. It is caused by irregular eating habits, emotional repression, excessive sexual intercourse.
'Empty irritation' is a condition which applies to the heart and is associated with Heat in the stomach. It is characterised by an unfulfilled desire to vomit, dizziness and anxiety. Jianshi stresses that the 'Empty' is 'hollow' rather than 'weak'. Nervous dyspepsia?

Section 2

INSOMNIA
H7 Sp6 Sp9 Sp1 Cx6 (A. Chamfrault)
B62 G41 L9
S36 T19 S27
B13 B30 G17
L1

29. PALPITATION OF THE HEART *ZHENG CHONG*

Section 1

CAUSE OF DISEASE	SYMPTOMS	DIAGNOSTIC FEATURES	MAIN POINTS	SECONDARY POINTS
1. Yin Empty and has little blood.	Heart agitated and palpitating.	Pulse Empty and Rapid.	Cv4 B15 H5 Cx7 S36	H7 Cv7 Cx6
2. Kidney water dried up and exhausted; heart Fire burns upwards.	Heart and Shen confused and disordered; heart agitated and palpitating; continuous discomfort waking and sleeping.	Pulse Rapid; tongue deep red.	H7 Cx6 H5 B15 B23	Cx7 S36 G35 S41

Section 2

PALPITATIONS
H7 H3 B15
Cx6
K24 K25
Cv12 Liv13
B10 G20

TACHYCARDIA
H5 Gv11 Gv14
G20 B10
Liv2
B38 B39 B13

ANGINA PECTORIS
K5 T7 Cv3
S36 B17 K2 Cv12 S19

ANGINA PECTORIS—cont.
Sp6 H8 Cx8 H3 G41
Cx1 Cx7 Si1 B60 B42

HYPERCHOLESTEROLAEMIA
Liv2

CARDIAC ASTHMA
H9 H4
Si14 Si15
L1 L2
Gv17 Cv18

ANAEMIA
B38 S36
L9 Sp5

30. AMNESIA *JIAN WANG*

Section 1

CAUSE OF DISEASE	SYMPTOMS	DIAGNOSTIC FEATURES	MAIN POINTS	SECONDARY POINTS
1. Kidney Empty; Knowledge deficient; heart Empty; Shen not filled up; heart and kidney both Empty; Fire and Water have not passed into their respective organs.	Shen and Si scattered; patient forgets what has happened.	Foot and Inch Pulses Empty.	B15 B23 Cv4 S36	H7 H3

CAUSE OF DISEASE	SYMPTOMS	DIAGNOSTIC FEATURES	MAIN POINTS	SECONDARY POINTS
2. Phlegm set in motion by Fire and covers the pericardium.	Shen Zhi confused.	Pulse Slippery; tongue greasy.	Cv12 S40 B15 S36	L7 H7 Cx6 K1

Section 2

AMNESIA
H9 H7 H3 Gv11 B15 B38 B39
Cx9 L3 Li11
Gv20
K1

31. LIVER WIND *GAN FENG*

Section 1

CAUSE OF DISEASE	SYMPTOMS	DIAGNOSTIC FEATURES	MAIN POINTS	SECONDARY POINTS
1. Yin deficient and has little blood; extreme Heat generates Wind.	Head and eyes dizzy; may have headache and tinnitus; muscular spasms.	Tongue deep red and not furred; Pulse Wiry, Fine and Rapid.	G20 B18 Cx6	G34 Liv2 Liv3
2. Violent anger; Qi anxious.	Patient suddenly collapses and becomes unconscious; teeth tightly clenched; face blue-green.	Pulse Wiry and has strength.	Gv20 Gv26 Cv12 XA1 (let blood)	Li4 Liv3 B54

32. HEADACHE *TOU TONG*

Section 1

CAUSE OF DISEASE	SYMPTOMS	DIAGNOSTIC FEATURES	MAIN POINTS	SECONDARY POINTS
1. Affected by Wind Evil.	Headache; dislikes the wind; nose blocked.	Pulse Floating; tongue thinly furred white.	Gv16 B12 Gv23 S8	Li4 T5 Li20
2. Affected by Cold Evil.	Headache; dislikes the cold; no sweating.	Pulse Floating and Tight.	as above	Li4 T5
3. Phlegm obstructs the Pure Yang.	Head dizzy and painful; vomiting and dizziness.	Pulse Wiry and Slowed-down; tongue furred and slippery.	G20 S8 Gv20	S40 Cx6 S36
4. Fire depressed and attacks upwards.	Head extremely painful; teeth also painful.	Pulse Wiry and Rapid; sides of tongue deep red.	XH3 (let blood) G20 Li4	Liv2

CAUSE OF DISEASE	SYMPTOMS	DIAGNOSTIC FEATURES	MAIN POINTS	SECONDARY POINTS
5. Weariness injures Qi	Headache; body weary; dyspnoea; little appetite.	Pulse Empty and Large; tongue pale.	Gv20 XH2 (or Gv24.5) B10	S36 Cv6
6. Yin blood deficient and damaged.	Continuous headache.	Pulse Hollow; pain in Fish Tail (?).	T23 B17 B18	XH3 S36
7. Side of head painful; Qi and blood Empty; liver Wind rebels.	Lateral headache; pain intermittent; headache continues intermittently all day.	Pulse Deep and Wiry.	G20 S8 T23 T3 G41	XH3 G14 S2 Li20 S7 Gv26
8. Phlegm and Heat attack upwards.	Left or right lateral headache (but consistently on one side, in contrast with 9).	Pulse Rapid or Slippery; tongue red, furred and greasy.	G20 S8 XH3 Cv12	L7 S40
9. Wind Evil invades the Luo.	Pain alternately severe and mild; may occur on either side of head.	Pulse Floating.	G20 G5 G4 B54	T5 G34

Section 2

HEADACHE, MIGRAINE
Hepatic type migraine — Liv8 G40
Fear and tension type — K5 L6
Feeling of heat — Sp2 Liv2 K2 S44
Many headaches or migraines respond to the first two of the above three groups.
    Other points, including localised points are often also needed:
G20 B10 Gv16
B2 G1 T17 T18 G12 G11 G10
L7 Si3 Si5
Pain in the temporal area is often due to liver and gall bladder.
Pain on the vertex is often due to kidney or bladder.
Supraorbital pain is often due to stomach or bladder.
Head heavy, tension: triple warmer.
Congestive headache: B62
Alcoholic hangover: G8 (S. de Morant).
S36 T12 Si1 B60 B57 G3 G4 G5 G6 Gv4 B22 Gv10
S41 G18 Cv4 Gv23 H3 B9 S1 S2 S3 S4 B12
B63 Gv18 Gv28 Li11 Si11 Li1
Li4 H7 Cv5 Gv20 S36 K1 B54 S8 G20

33. VERTIGO *XUAN YUN*

Section 1

CAUSE OF DISEASE	SYMPTOMS	DIAGNOSTIC FEATURES	MAIN POINTS	SECONDARY POINTS
1. Phlegm and Fire depressed in Upper Warmer; Wind Evil ascends into the Qiao Luo.	Head and eyes dizzy.	Both Inch Pulses Empty and Large; sides of tongue deep red.	Gv20 G20 S8 Li4	XH3 CX7 Liv3
2. Yin Empty; Fire brilliant; Water dried up; Fire ascends.	Dizziness; heart troubled.	Both Foot Pulses Empty and Rapid; mouth dry.	Cv4 B23	S36 K6
3. Phlegm-fluid rebels upwards.	Dizziness; desire to vomit.	Pulse Wiry and Slippery; tongue furred, slippery and greasy; mouth glutinous; no thirst.	Gv20 Cv12 G20 Li4 Gv23	G34 S40 S36 S41
4. Liver Fire rushes upwards.	Dizziness; quick tempered and prone to anger.	Left Connecting Pulse Wiry and Full.	Gv20 G20 B18 H7 K1	Li4 Liv3 G34 K6

Section 2

VERTIGO
Li4 S40 G20
B16 Gv20 B62 B67 B8
Gv23 G20 Cx1 Gv19
Si3 B62 Si7
B66

SYNCOPE
Li10 Gv26
L9 T2 Liv1
H9 Cx9

SYNCOPE—cont.
Sp6 G43 S45
B57

CEREBRAL CONGESTION
K1 B62
Li1 L11
S36 Cx7

MENINGISM
B62 S13

34. INTERCOSTAL NEURALGIA *XIE TONG*

Section 1

CAUSE OF DISEASE	SYMPTOMS	DIAGNOSTIC FEATURES	MAIN POINTS	SECONDARY POINTS
1. Left ribs painful: dead blood in ribs.	Left ribs painful; pain does not move.	Pulse Wiry and Rough; tongue substance dark purple.	Liv14 Liv13 B17 B18	Cx6 Liv4

CAUSE OF DISEASE	SYMPTOMS	DIAGNOSTIC FEATURES	MAIN POINTS	SECONDARY POINTS
2. Right ribs painful: Phlegm stopped up; Qi obstructed.	Right ribs swollen and painful; pleuritic rub.	Pulse Wiry and Slippery; tongue furred, slippery and white.	Liv14 (rt.h.side) B18 Cv12 Cv17	Cx6 (rt.h.side) S40 (lt.h.side) G40 (lt.h.side) Sp17 (rt.h.side)
3. Liver Full: liver brilliant; Qi rebels.	Ribs on both sides painful; difficult to turn the body.	Pulse Deep, Wiry and has strength; face blue-green.	Liv14 B18 Liv13	T6 G34 Cx6 Liv3
4. Liver Empty: liver Empty and depressed, rebels.	Slight pain in ribs on both sides; pain extends to shoulders and chest.	Pulse Wiry and Empty.	Cv14 Liv13 Liv14 B18	Cx6 G40 K6
5. Liver Hot: liver meridian Full and Hot.	Ribs on both sides painful; heart troubled, anxious and prone to anger; constipation; urine yellow.	Pulse Full and Rapid; tongue yellow and greasy; tinnitus.	Liv14 Liv13 B18 Cv3	T6 G34 S36
6. Food stopped up: food and drink obstructed.	Taste in mouth foul and sour; stomach obstructed and full; dislikes food.	Pulse Deep and Slippery; tongue thickly furred.	Liv14 Liv13 Cv12 S25	Cx6 Sp4 G34 S36

Section 2

INTERCOSTAL NEURALGIA
L9 Li4 B13
B17 Liv13 Cv17
G41 S36 Si5
T6 B62 K1

35. NUMBNESS including Rheumatism and similar conditions   *BI ZHENG*

Section 1

CAUSE OF DISEASE	SYMPTOMS	DIAGNOSTIC FEATURES	MAIN POINTS	SECONDARY POINTS
1. Moving numbness: Wind, Cold and Damp Qi lodge in meridians; Wind exceeds Cold and Damp.	Wind Evil flows up and down, fighting with the Good Qi in places where it is Empty; muscles flaccid; pain does not occur in any fixed place.	1. Wind Evil attacks Damp and moves into the four limbs and shoulders; Pulse Floating, Rough and Tight.	Gv14 Li15 Li11 G31 G34	T5 B58 Li4 B54

CAUSE OF DISEASE	SYMPTOMS	DIAGNOSTIC FEATURES	MAIN POINTS	SECONDARY POINTS
		2. Limb joints swollen and painful; pain never ceases.	G39	
2. Painful numbness: Cold exceeds Wind and Damp.	Limbs cramped and painful; severe if cold, relieved if warm.	1. Occurs only at night; pain like the bite of a tiger (this is called the 'White Tiger passing through the joints Wind); Pulse Rough and Tight. 2. If associated with Damp it occurs in dull (i.e. Yin) weather; body feels heavy.	Li15 Li11 Li4 G31 G34 B19 B20	T5 G38 Sp6
3. Summer-heat numbness: Damp exceeds Wind and Cold.	Painful and does not shift; heavy sweating; limbs slow and weak; Jing Shen confused and obstructed; skin numb.	1. Numb as though Insect moving in the flesh, unlike itching or pain. Empty Qi is the Root, Wind and Phlegm are the Signs (Note 1). 2. Does not itch, is not painful; not sensitive when pressed or pinched; it is like the solidity of wood; dead blood congeals and forms blockage; Wind and Cold attack outside.	Cv12 Cv6 S36 B17 B20 B23 Li11 G34	B12 T5 B53 Sp6

NOTES

1. *Empty Qi is the principal cause of the condition, Wind and Phlegm are the 'external manifestations', the secondary contributary factors.*

Section 2

RHEUMATIC DISEASES
Muscular or early arthritic.
Often the Luo point on the opposite side is useful i.e.: Very early osteo-arthritis of the right hip, with pain going down lateral side of leg (gall bladder meridian) and inside groin (kidney meridian). Use K6 left and G37 left. Brachial neuralgia on right, with pain along course of small intestine meridian. Use Si7 left and possibly local points such as G20 G21 T15.
Pain base of thumb. Use L7 and Li6 on opposite side, with possibly L9 and Li5 on same side. Sprained knee, with pain behind knee, and on either side of patella. Use B58 Sp4 G40 on opposite side.
Damaged ring finger or early rheumatism. T5 on opposite side.
Category III points may be used.
The above, and other, basic principles may be used in any part of the body.

LUMBAGO, SCIATICA
K5 B62 B54
B23 K5 Cx9
Gv4 B28 B48 B49
B31 to 35

NUMBNESS
Cx8 H3

36. NUMBNESS OF THE CHEST *XIONG BI*

Section 1

CAUSE OF DISEASE	SYMPTOMS	DIAGNOSTIC FEATURES	MAIN POINTS	SECONDARY POINTS
1. Yang Qi in chest does not move; Yin Evil ascends.	Dyspnoea; coughing; chest and back painful; chest blocked and melancholy.	Inch Pulse Deep and Slow; superficial Connecting Pulse Small, Tight and Rapid; tongue furred white.	Gv12 Gv10 B13 Cv17 Cx6	L5 Cv12 S36
2. Yang Qi in chest does not move; Phlegm-fluid rebels upwards.	Chest numb; cannot sleep; whole of chest and back painful; noise in chest.	Pulse Deep, Wiry, Minute and Slippery, or Deep and Slippery.	Cv12 Liv13 Cx6 B17 B13	
3. Cold and rebellious Qi in chest attacks upwards.	Chest blocked and full; region below the heart rebels against the heart.	Pulse Deep and Full.	B16 B17 Liv13 Cx6 Cv17	

Section 2

See other pulmonary and cardiac diseases:
Nos. 3, 5, 22, 29.

37. PARALYSIS *WEI*

Section 1

CAUSE OF DISEASE	SYMPTOMS	DIAGNOSTIC FEATURES	MAIN POINTS	SECONDARY POINTS
1. Damp and Heat: affected by Seasonal Damp and Heat.	Both legs paralysed and weak; limbs extremely weary.	Pulse Weak-floating and Rapid; face pale and yellow; tongue furred white and slippery; head heavy.	S30 S36 G30 G39 G34	B20 G20
2. Damp and Heat flow downwards; Damp in Lower Warmer overflowing.	Both feet paralysed and weak; fever; urine red; polyuria.	Pulse Deep and Slippery; tongue furred and greasy; mouth glutinous.	as above	Sp6 K6 Gv16

CAUSE OF DISEASE	SYMPTOMS	DIAGNOSTIC FEATURES	MAIN POINTS	SECONDARY POINTS
3. Yin Empty and associated with Damp and Heat.	Legs have no strength to move; feet hot.	Pulse Fine and Rapid; tongue dry; heart troubled.	as above	K6 Sp10 Gv16
4. Chronic disease in which Qi and blood are Empty and weak.	Both legs paralysed and weak; dyspnoea; spontaneous sweating.	Six Pulses Empty and Pliable; tongue pale; face paralysed and yellow.	as above	B20 B21
5. Liver and kidney Empty and damaged.	Muscles and bones paralysed and weak; cannot walk.	Pulses in both feet Fine and Weak; tongue pale; ₋o Shen; flesh wasted away.	as above	B23 B18 B11

Section 2 WEAKNESS OF LEGS
S35 XL2
G30 G41
K2 K10

38. DIABETES (see Note 1) *XIAO KE*

Section 1

CAUSE OF DISEASE	SYMPTOMS	DIAGNOSTIC FEATURES	MAIN POINTS	SECONDARY POINTS
1. Upper Wasting: lung meridian Dry and Hot.	Excessive drinking, micturition normal.	Right Inch Pulse Large; face red; tongue furred yellow.	B13 B15	Cx6 L10
2. Middle Wasting: stomach Dry and Hot.	Thirsty; good appetite; emaciated.	Right Connecting Pulse Overflowing and Rapid; tongue red and furred yellow; constipated.	B21 Cv12	K3 S44
3. Lower Wasting: kidney Yin Empty and dried up.	Thirsty; micturition immediately after drinking; limbs emaciated.	Both Foot Pulses without strength; feet and shins painful and weak.	B15 B23 Cv4 Cv3	K7 B60

NOTES
1. *The heading of the disease is literally 'wasting and thirst' which the Cihai gives as an old term for the Chinese word now used for 'diabetes'.*

39. GOITRE *YING QI*

Section 1

CAUSE OF DISEASE	SYMPTOMS	DIAGNOSTIC FEATURES	MAIN POINTS	SECONDARY POINTS
Qi obstructed, blood	Large hard swelling on neck.	Does not move when	appropriate	G21

CAUSE OF DISEASE	SYMPTOMS	DIAGNOSTIC FEATURES	MAIN POINTS	SECONDARY POINTS
congealed; Phlegm and Heat may be congealed.		pressed; no pain when touched.	local points.	T10 Toxic Goitre:
				1. With palpitations of the heart Cx6 H7
				2. With heavy sweating Li4
				3. With swollen eyes B1 B2 S2 G20
				4. With high blood-pressure Gv20

40. SPONTANEOUS SWEATING   *ZI HAN*

Section 1

CAUSE OF DISEASE	SYMPTOMS	DIAGNOSTIC FEATURES	MAIN POINTS	SECONDARY POINTS
1. Exterior Yin Empty.	Sweating not due to natural causes such as wearing thick clothes in hot weather, or strenuous movement.	Sweating for no reason.	Gv14 Cv4 B38 B23	Li4 K7 S36
2. Wei Yang not strong, Wind Evil affects the Wei, Wei Qi cannot keep it out, so the skin becomes slow and the pores flaccid; as a result of this, Fluid pours wildly out of the skin.	Fluid moves wildly and pours out of the body.	For no reason sweat pours out of the body.	Gv14 Cv4	Li4 S44
3. Body fat; pores dilated; Sunlight Yang Hot.	Sweating for no reason.	Intermittent spontaneous sweating.	Cv12 S36	Li4 S44

EXCESSIVE PERSPIRATION	LACK OF PERSPIRATION
L11 Sp15 B17 T10 Gv16	L8 Sp2 Li4
B13 H7	G11 G44
B62	Cx9 S43 S45
	Li1 Li4 Si2 L8

41. NOCTURNAL SWEATING   *DAO HAN*

Section 1

CAUSE OF DISEASE	SYMPTOMS	DIAGNOSTIC FEATURES	MAIN POINTS	SECONDARY POINTS
Yin is Empty and cannot stimulate its Mai Qi outside the body (Note 1); Fluid cannot be restrained; during sleep the Wei Qi activates the Yin, blood and Qi have nothing on which to rely for support, so the pores open and sweat is emitted.	Sweating when asleep; sweating ceases on waking.	Sweating when asleep.	Gv14 H6 Si3 B13 Cv6 Cv4	Cv7 Sp6

NOTES
1. *Mai Qi: the Qi which pertains to the Mai or blood-vessels.*

Section 2

NOCTURNAL SWEATING
L1
Cv6 B15 H7
K2
Si3 K7 T5 (S. de Morant)

42. RECTAL BLEEDING   *BIAN XUE*

Section 1

CAUSE OF DISEASE	SYMPTOMS	DIAGNOSTIC FEATURES	MAIN POINTS	SECONDARY POINTS
1. Near blood: large intestine Damp and Hot.	Blood passed through rectum; blood visible before stools.	Pulse Deep and Rapid; urine red.	B25 Gv1 B57	B35
2. Distant blood: small intestine Cold and Damp.	Blood passed through rectum; stools visible before blood.	Pulse Deep and Slowed-down; urine white.	Sp1 S36	B27 (moxa) Sp6

CAUSE OF DISEASE	SYMPTOMS	DIAGNOSTIC FEATURES	MAIN POINTS	SECONDARY POINTS
3. Intestine Wind: blood in large intestine Hot and affected by Wind.	Blood passed through rectum; blood thin and bright.	Both Foot Pulses Floating.	B25 Gv1 B57	B17
4. Damp and Heat collect poison.	Blood passed through rectum; blood thick and dark.	Both Foot Pulses Slippery.	Gv1 B57 B20 B23	Sp10 B17

Section 2

HAEMORRHOIDS
B58 B57 B54
Gv1 B35 B47 B48 B49
Liv8 Cx7
Sp5 G39
K5 K8 K10 B50
Gv20 B60

43. EPISTAXIS *NU XUE*

Section 1

CAUSE OF DISEASE	SYMPTOMS	DIAGNOSTIC FEATURES	MAIN POINTS	SECONDARY POINTS
1. Fire pursues, blood rebels.	Sudden bleeding from nose with great force.	Pulse Overflowing and Slippery; blood purple; face red.	Li4 Gv23 Gv14 Gv16	Li20 Gv26 XH2 B64
2. Qi Empty, blood not strong.	Bleeding from nose continues intermittently for whole day.	Pulse Hollow and without strength; blood light red; face hoary-white.	B20 Sp1 Cv13	Gv23 B17 S36
3. Wind and Cold obstructed and overflow into meridians; blood moves wildly.	Dislikes the cold; fever; headache; no sweating.	Pulse Floating and Tight; tongue furred white.	Gv23 Gv16 Gv14 B12	Li4 G20
4. Interior of body Empty and Cold; upper part of body False and Hot.	Nose bleeds all day long; not stopped by Cool Medicine.	Pulse Hollow and Slowed-down or Empty and Fine; tongue pale; mouth dry but no wish to drink.	Gv14 B20 (moxa)	Cv4 (moxa) S36

Section 2

EPISTAXIS
Liv5 Si1 B18
Gv24 Gv20 Gv15 Li19
G21 Si15 G20 B10

EPISTAXIS—cont.
Li11 Li10 Li4 S44
Cv4 B54 S36
Si2 L3 G39 B64 Liv1

44. INTERNAL WEAKNESS *LONG BI*

Section 1

CAUSE OF DISEASE	SYMPTOMS	DIAGNOSTIC FEATURES	MAIN POINTS	SECONDARY POINTS
1. Heat congealed below.	Hot feeling in abdomen; stools hard.	Pulse Deep and Full; tongue furred yellow.	Cv4 Cv3 B23 B28 B22	Liv8 Sp9 Sp6 K1
2. Yang Empty.	Dislikes the cold.	Pulse Empty and Fine; tongue furred pale and white.	Cv4 Cv3 B20 B23	S36 Sp6
3. Yin Empty.	Fever after midday; mouth parched; tongue burning.	Pulse Empty and Wiry.	Cv4 Sp6 Cv3	Cx7 Sp9 Li4
4. Middle Qi deficient.	Abdomen not anxious or full; extremely weary; dyspnoea; no Strength in speech.	Pulse Empty and Weak.	Cv6 Cv4 B38 B20	S36 Sp6

Section 2

RETENTION OF URINE	PROSTATIC HYPERTROPHY
Cv6 Cv4 K2 K11	B67 K3
Sp9 Sp10	Cv2 Cv3 Cv4
Li9 S37 B54	Sp9 Sp10

45. INTERMITTENT SWELLINGS (Note 1) *SHAN QI*

Section 1

CAUSE OF DISEASE	SYMPTOMS	DIAGNOSTIC FEATURES	MAIN POINTS	SECONDARY POINTS
1. Rushing Swelling: liver Evil rebels upwards.	Lower abdomen painful; Qi rushes upwards to the heart; constipation and dysuria.	Pulse Deep, Wiry and Tight; face blue-green.	B23 Cv4 Liv3	Sp6 K6
2. Lonely Swelling: Cold and Damp invade testicles.	When lying down the testicles retract, when standing up they descend.	Pulse Deep and Wiry.	Cv3 Liv1 B23	S29 Sp6
3. Tui Swelling: Cold and Damp congealed in scrotum.	Scrotum swollen and large.	Pulse Hard.	B23 Cv6 Cv4	Sp9 Liv1

CAUSE OF DISEASE	SYMPTOMS	DIAGNOSTIC FEATURES	MAIN POINTS	SECONDARY POINTS
4. Cold Swelling: spleen receives liver Evil.	Lower abdomen painful; desire to vomit.	Pulse Deep and Tight.	B23 Cv4	Liv2 S36
5. Gui Swelling: dead blood congeals and forms abscess.	Lower abdomen swollen on both sides like a cucumber.	Pulse Deep and Slippery.	Cv4 Cv3 Sp10	Liv1 T5
6. Swelling of small intestine: Wind and Cold invade small intestine.	Pain in lower abdomen extending to testicles.	Foot Pulse Wiry and Tight.	Cv4 B23	K6 Liv3
7. Bladder Qi: Cold congeals in bladder.	Lower abdomen swollen and painful; unable to micturate.	Pulse Deep and Slow.	B23 Cv3	Liv8 Sp6

NOTES

1. *The heading is a combination of what is now a common term for 'hernia', Shan, plus the ubiquitous Qi. But although hernia is probably represented here, it is difficult to reconcile all the above symptoms with herniae alone. Moreover none of the Chinese definitions of Shan specifically refer to any 'protrusion' (Tu Chu).*
Jianshi gives: 'Acute pain in testicles and lower abdomen; may be greater on one side than the other. Scrotum swollen, pain generally over whole area; if severe, abdomen is gathered like a cup or a bowl.'
Cıhai gives: 'The Su Wen says: "Pain in lower abdomen, inability to micturate or defaecate". Yin Qi accumulates inside the body, Cold Qi in the abdomen causes Ying and Wei to be out of harmony (see Introduction), blood and Qi to be Empty and Weak; thus Cold Wind enters the abdomen and causes Shan. There are many varieties of Shan.' The scant definitions of these 'many varieties' provide no more information than is given above as symptoms. Nos. 3 and 4, Tui, and Gui, have no meanings other than types of Shan.

46. INCONTINENCE OF URINE *YI NIAO*

Section 1

CAUSE OF DISEASE	SYMPTOMS	DIAGNOSTIC FEATURES	MAIN POINTS	SECONDARY POINTS
1. Bladder Empty and Cold.	Incontinence of urine which is passed without cause.	Both Foot Pulses Deep and Fine; face withered and dark.	B23 B28 Cv6 Cv4 Cv3	Sp9 Sp6 Liv1
2. Bladder Empty and Hot.	Incontinence of urine which is passed without cause.	Both Foot Pulses Fine and Rapid; urine red.	Cv6 Cv4 Cv3 B23 B28	B24 Sp9 Sp6

INCONTINENCE OF URINE	NOCTURNAL ENURESIS
B67 Cv1 Sp9 B27 B28	K10
S36 L7 L9	
Gv4 T4	

47. URETHRAL DISCHARGE (Note 1)   *CHI BAI ZHUO*

Section 1

CAUSE OF DISEASE	SYMPTOMS	DIAGNOSTIC FEATURES	MAIN POINTS	SECONDARY POINTS
1. White discharge: Lower Warmer Damp and Hot.	Thick purulent discharge; sometimes purulent matter remains in urethra.	Pulse Deep and Slippery; mouth glutinous and greasy.	B23 Cv6 Cv4 Liv13	Liv8 Sp6 K6 Sp4
2. Red discharge: Damp and Heat injure the blood.	Sometimes red purulent matter in urethra.	Pulse Deep and Rapid; mouth parched; heart troubled; restless sleep.	B15 B23 B28 H8 Cv4	Sp9 Sp6

NOTES

1. *The Chinese heading literally means 'red and white turbid-fluid'. Confusion arises since 'white turbid-fluid' is a modern word for 'gonorrhoea', but so too is Lin, the heading of the next section, No. 48. This problem is not really solved by omitting 'gonorrhoea' from both headings, as has been done; but it is certainly far safer to rely on the symptoms given, rather than on a possibly inaccurate modern equivalent for an old Chinese term.*

Section 2

URETHRITIS
B31 B32 B33 B34 B35
Cv1 K11
K9 K10 Sp6
S25 S28 Cv4 Cv12 Liv1

48. URINARY DISEASES (see Notes to No. 47)   *LIN*

Section 1

CAUSE OF DISEASE	SYMPTOMS	DIAGNOSTIC FEATURES	MAIN POINTS	SECONDARY POINTS
1. Qi leakage: Transforming action of Qi not effective.	Retention of urine with overflow; lower abdomen full and painful.	Pulse Deep and Wiry and without strength.	Cv4 Cv3 B23 B24	Cv6 Sp9 K6 S28 Sp6

CAUSE OF DISEASE	SYMPTOMS	DIAGNOSTIC FEATURES	MAIN POINTS	SECONDARY POINTS
2. Blood leakage: blood depressed in bladder.	Blood in urine; urethra painful; incessant urge to micturate.	Pulse Deep and Rough; tongue substance deep red; heart troubled; mouth parched.	Cv4 Cv3 Sp10 B23 B27	K7 B54 Sp9 Sp6
3. Stone leakage: bladder stores Heat.	Urine concentrated and contains gravel; penis painful during micturition	Pulse Wiry and Anxious; micturition incessant	Cv4 Cv3 B23 B22 B27	B28 S28 B54 K1
4. Grease leakage: kidney Empty.	Urine like grease; micturition painful.	Foot Pulse Empty and Pliable.	Cv6 Cv4 Cv3 B23 B22	Sp9 Sp6 B28 Cv5
5. Weariness leakage: great weariness injures spleen.	Slight and painful urinary incontinence, occurring when weary.	Pulse Empty; face yellow; dyspnoea; limbs weak	Cv6 Cv4 Cv3 B20 B23 B22	Sp9 Sp6 K6 Li4 L5

Section 2

NEPHRITIS
K5 B54
B22 B23 B24 B62
Cv3 S36 Sp14
G24 G25

CYSTITIS
B26 B27 B28 B29 B30
B54 Cv2 K12 Sp6 G25
S30 S31 Liv11 Gv1

49 SPERMATORRHOEA (see Note 1) *YI JING*

Section 1

CAUSE OF DISEASE	SYMPTOMS	DIAGNOSTIC FEATURES	MAIN POINTS	SECONDARY POINTS
1. Sovereign and Minister Fires (i.e. heart and kidney) blaze brightly and burn the Yin.	Nocturnal emissions after dreaming.	Inch and Foot Pulses Overflowing or Rapid; mouth dry; urine red.	B15 B23 Cv4 Cv3	H7 Sp6 K12
2. Heart and kidney deficient.	Nocturnal emissions without dreams; associated with palpitation of the heart, vertigo and aching of legs.	Inch and Foot Pulses Deep, Weak and without strength; face appears emaciated.	B15 B23 B38 Cv4	K12 S36 Sp6

CAUSE OF DISEASE	SYMPTOMS	DIAGNOSTIC FEATURES	MAIN POINTS	SECONDARY POINTS
3. Mental anxiety injures the spleen.	Nocturnal emissions; palpitation of the heart; insomnia; loss of appetite; general feeling of weakness.	Pulse Empty and Slowed-down; face haggard.	B38 B44 B42 B20 B23	H7 S36 Sp6
4. Accumulated Thoughts (Si: see Introduction) not coordinated.	Intermittent loss of sperm; Shen and Si confused.	Pulse Empty and Floating.	H7 Cv4 B23 B47	B32 Cv3 Sp6
5. Excessive sexual activity; Sperm Barrier weak.	Continuous leakage of sperm which patient cannot control; head dizzy; feet weak; Jing Shen wasted and withered.	Pulse Fine and without strength.	B23 B47 B38 Cv4 Cv3	K12 S36 Sp6
6. Damp and Heat of spleen and stomach remain dormant in the Yin.	Intermittent loss of sperm; mouth greasy; no appetite.	Pulse Deep and Slippery; body fat; tongue thickly furred and greasy.	Cv12 B20 B21	Cv2 Sp9 S36

NOTES

1. *For the Chinese theory of the composition, function etc. of Sperm (Jing), see Introduction.*

Section 2

SPERMATORRHOEA
Sp6
Cv4 Cv3
S36 S25
B31 B32 B33 B34
K23 B47 Sp9

SPERMATORRHOEA—cont.
B67 K12

NYMPHOMANIA
Sp20 S30 S29
Liv2 K3 G43

50. IMPOTENCE   *YANG WEI*

Section 1

CAUSE OF DISEASE	SYMPTOMS	DIAGNOSTIC FEATURES	MAIN POINTS	SECONDARY POINTS
1. Excessive sexual desire.	Penis unable to become erect. Secondary symptoms: loins painful; legs ache.	Foot Pulse Empty and without strength.	B38 B18 B23 Gv3 Cv4	S36 Sp6 G34 Liv3

CAUSE OF DISEASE	SYMPTOMS	DIAGNOSTIC FEATURES	MAIN POINTS	SECONDARY POINTS
2. Anxieties depressed and congealed, injure heart and spleen.	As above. Secondary symptoms: Jing Energy exhausted; no appetite; face appears withered and yellow.	Pulse Slowed-down and Weak.	B38 B20 B21 Cv4	Li10
3. Repression injures liver.	As above. Secondary symptoms: Jing Shen upset; chest melancholy and uncomfortable.	(no observations)	Liv13 B18 Cv3	Cv11 Cx6 Liv5 Liv3
4. Damp overflowing, body flourishing.	As above.	Tongue furred white and greasy; pulse Weak-floating and Slippery.	B20 B23 Cv3	S36 (moxa) S28 Sp9
5. Damp and Heat flow downwards.	As above. Secondary symptoms: testicles cold; emits Yin sweat; urine yellowish-red and foul smelling.	(no observations)	S28 K12 Cv3	Sp9 K7 Liv2

Section 2

IMPOTENCE
K10 K2 Liv4 Liv1
S30 Sp6 Cv6
Gv4 K3 L7
K12 Cv2

LACK OF DESIRE
T4 Gv1 Gv2
Liv8 Si5

LACK OF DESIRE—cont.
Cv5 Cv6 S28 S45

FRIGIDITY
K7
Cv4 Cv7
Cv1
S29 Sp6

51. RED AND WHITE SORES   *CHI BAI YOU FENG*

Section 1

CAUSE OF DISEASE	SYMPTOMS	DIAGNOSTIC FEATURES	MAIN POINTS	SECONDARY POINTS
1. Red sores: spleen and lungs Dry and Hot; caused by struggle between the blood and the Wind Evil which has invaded the blood.	Skin develops red patches which may occur anywhere on the body; the patches are swollen and puffy, inflamed and hot, painful and itching.	Pulse Floating and Rapid.	B12 Li11	B54 Sp10

CAUSE OF DISEASE	SYMPTOMS	DIAGNOSTIC FEATURES	MAIN POINTS	SECONDARY POINTS
2. White sores: spleen and lungs Dry and Hot; caused by struggle between Qi and the Wind Evil which has invaded Qi.	Skin develops white patches which may occur anywhere on the body; the patches are swollen and puffy, inflamed and hot, painful and itching.	Pulse Floating.	Li11 T5	B58 G31

52. DAMP RASH *SHI ZHEN*

Section 1

CAUSE OF DISEASE	SYMPTOMS	DIAGNOSTIC FEATURES	MAIN POINTS	SECONDARY POINTS
Wind Damp, blood Hot	Eruption of small white pustules over whole body.	Itching; sudden rise in temperature; pustules emit yellow fluid when broken.	Li11 B54 Sp10	Li15 T5 Li4

53. RASH (?) *PEI LEI*

Section 1

Affected by Wind when sweating or by Cold when sleeping uncovered; Wind Evil enters the skin.	At first skin itches, then develops pimples like the two halves of a bean; body slightly hot; body itches; heart troubled.	Pulse Floating.	Li11 T5 B54 B13	Sp10 G31

Section 2

PURPLISH DISCOLOURATION OF FACE
L9

PRURITIS
Liv8 B54
B13 S15
G41 L7
G37 G31 Gv20

ACNE VULGARIS
L11 H9
Sp2 B54
Liv11 K12

URTICARIA
Liv5 Li14
Sp6 S31

FURUNCULOSIS
L11 H9
plus deep breathing.

WEEPING ECZEMA
B60 B54 Li11
T5 Si3 Sp10

54. SORES IN MOUTH, DEGENERATIVE DISEASES OF MOUTH, THRUSH
KOU CHUANG, KOU MI, E KOU CHUANG

Section 1

CAUSE OF DISEASE	SYMPTOMS	DIAGNOSTIC FEATURES	MAIN POINTS	SECONDARY POINTS
1. Empty Fire: excessive mental anxiety; heart and kidney not connected; Empty Fire burns upwards.	Mouth develops pale sores; interior of mouth heavily streaked and mottled white; in severe cases mucosa comes off in patches.	Pulse Empty; no thirst.	B15 B23 Cv24 Li4	B27 S36 K6 B20
2. Full Fire: excessive eating and excessive drinking of alcohol cause the Full Fire of the heart to move wildly.	Mouth develops bright red sores; whole mouth rotten and mottled; in severe cases the jaw and tongue are swollen.	Pulse Full; mouth dry.	Li4 S36 B15 B20	Cv24 H8 Sp2 XM2 (lt.h.side) XM2 (rt.h.side) (let blood)
3. Full Fire: excessive eating of rich foods; Full Heat obstructed and overflowing.	Whole mouth rotten and destroyed; in severe cases spreads to throat; cannot eat or drink; mouth foul smelling; constipation.	Mouth parched; Pulse Full.	Li4 Cv12 S36 Cx7	H8 Cv24 Liv2 S44 XM2 (both sides; let blood)
4. Empty Fire: body may be weak after long illness.	Whole mouth rotten and decayed; face haggard; sleep extremely agitated; Shen Qi diminished.	Pulse Slow and Sloweddown; mouth dry, little thirst.	Li4 S36 B20 B21	Cv12 Cv6 Sp6
5. Spleen Yang Empty and weak: spleen Qi Empty, Yang Qi weary.	Whole mouth rotten and decayed; loose motions; rumblings in abdomen; limbs weak; breathing shallow; face greenish-white.	Pulse Slow and Sloweddown.	Li4 S36 S25	Cv12 Cv6 B20 B21 Sp6
6. Minister Fire (kidney) moves wildly; over indulgence, lack of self-control; kidney Empty; little Jing Energy.	Whole mouth rotten and decayed; throat dry and burning; hands and heart troubled and hot.	Pulse Fine and Rapid.	Li4 K6 B23	Cv24 Cx7 T2

CAUSE OF DISEASE	SYMPTOMS	DIAGNOSTIC FEATURES	MAIN POINTS	SECONDARY POINTS
7. Pregnant womb Heat attacks upwards.	Whole mouth develops painful white spots; in severe cases the throat is swollen; difficulty in breast-feeding; patient weeps frequently.	Pulse Rapid; lines on the fingers purple.	Li4 S36	L11 Li1 (let blood) K3

Section 2	BITTER TASTE IN MOUTH G38 Liv5 S36	THRUSH Liv2 Cx8 K6
	LIPS CRACKED S4 Liv3 Li4 T5 G41	PAIN ROOT OF TONGUE Cv23 G20 H5 Cx7
	GLOSSITIS H9 Cx9 Li4 Cv24 Cv23 K2 Gv12 T5 G41	MOUTH DRY L5 Gv28 Liv8

55. TOOTHACHE *YA TONG*

Section 1

CAUSE OF DISEASE	SYMPTOMS	DIAGNOSTIC FEATURES	MAIN POINTS	SECONDARY POINTS
1. Fire depressed.	Gums swollen; whole of gums intermittently painful.	Pulse Rapid; tongue furred yellow; constipation.	Li4 S7 S6 S44	Li3 Gv26 Cv24
2. Affected by Wind.	Gums first swollen; if swelling continues then pain begins; pain severe when breathing in through mouth.	Pulse Floating; tongue thinly furred white.	as above	T17
3. Rich foods, Damp and Heat are Transformed into Teeth Worms. (Note 1).	Teeth eaten away by worms and collapse; if one tooth becomes rotten all the teeth will be eaten away; teeth ache continuously.	Tongue furred but appears normal; holes in teeth.	as above	
4. Kidney Empty.	Teeth loose and painful; if severe patient hates cold.	Both Foot Pulses without strength, or Rapid and Fine.	as above	K6

NOTES
1. *Certain diseases are traditionally attributed to 'Chong' i.e. 'worms' or 'insects'. In the past the removal of these Chong from the body was a specialised occupation.*

TOOTHACHE (Mainly neuralgia of teeth)   GINGIVITIS
G37 (opposite side to pain) G41   Gv28 S4 Li19
Li4 S44 S6   G16 Si8 L7
Li2 T23 T21 Gv26   Li3 S44 T9 S5
B60 B62   Gv27 T17
Cv24 B23 Li3

56. THROAT SWOLLEN AND PAINFUL   *YAN HOU ZHONG TONG*

Section 1

CAUSE OF DISEASE	SYMPTOMS	DIAGNOSTIC FEATURES	MAIN POINTS	SECONDARY POINTS
1. Affected by Seasonal Evil from outside.	Fever, dislikes the cold; throat swollen and painful; eating and drinking difficult; voice croaks.	Pulse Floating, and Rapid; right Inch and Connecting Pulses Abundant.	L11 (let blood) Li4 Gv16 L5	T1 Li1 (let blood) T5 Cv22
2. Full Fire: excessive eating of savoury foods; Hot Poison uneasy and congealed.	Throat swollen and painful; great thirst; constipation; phlegm hot, blocked and overflowing.	Pulse Full and Rapid; throat red and swollen.	L11 XM2 (both sides, let blood) Li4	T2 L10
3. Empty Fire: prone to anger; fond of drinking; likes wine and sex; causes Empty Fire to form obstruction in upper part of body.	Throat dry, tongue parched; heart troubled; mouth parched.	Pulse Empty and Rapid; throat painful but not severe; or pain may be severe where swollen.	K3 Li4 L5	S36 S44 Gv16

Section 2

TONSILLITIS
K5 Li4 Si17
L3 Li9 B12 Cv22
T10 G38 Si8
Li7 T2
S6 L11 Li5 Cx7
K1 Cv22 S40

PHARYNGITIS
L9 Li6
G20 B17 B18 Si14 S9 S10

PHARYNGITIS—cont.
Cv22 Cv23 T16 T15
S6 S5

LACK OF TASTE
Sp5 Sp4 S44

CERVICAL ADENITIS
B38 Si8 G41 T5
T10 H3 Li14 Li13
S12 Cv17 Cx1 Liv3

57. TINNITUS *ER MING*

Section 1

CAUSE OF DISEASE	SYMPTOMS	DIAGNOSTIC FEATURES	MAIN POINTS	SECONDARY POINTS
1. Gall-bladder Fire ascends; Wind and Cold restrained outside the body.	Continuous tinnitus.	Pulse Wiry and Rapid; face red; tongue dry; mouth bitter.	G20 Si19 T17	T5 G43 G34
2. Kidney Yin deficient; floating Heat ascends.	Tinnitus variable in intensity.	Pulse Rapid but without strength; mouth and tongue dry; tongue red and not furred.	Si19 K6	H3 K1

Section 2

TINNITUS
K1 G44
G20 B10
G7 G8 G9 G18 Gv16 Gv14
Catarrhal—Liv4 Si16 T17 Si19
L11 Li4 K3 S36
T5 G2 T21 Gv20 Gv19 T18
Si3 Si5 Si19 Si16

TINNITUS—cont.
B62 Cx7

OTITIS EXTERNA
G1 Si19 Li4 Li11

OVER-PRODUCTION OF CERUMEN
T17 T21 Si18 Li4

58. DEAFNESS *ER LONG*

Section 1

CAUSE OF DISEASE	SYMPTOMS	DIAGNOSTIC FEATURES	MAIN POINTS	SECONDARY POINTS
1. Gall-bladder Fire blazing and abundant, moves upwards into the empty spaces.	Sudden complete deafness.	Pulse Wiry; tongue red; heart troubled; prone to anger.	Si19 T17 B19	T5 G43
2. Kidney Yin deficient, cannot moisten the holes (of the head, i.e. including the ears).	Deafness which begins slowly and increases.	Shen exhausted; loins ache; face dark.	Not suitable for acupuncture	

Section 2

DEAFNESS
Li1 Cx9
T21 T23 T19
K8 K5

OTITIS MEDIA
T23 G1 Li4
T18 T19 G20
T17 G2

DEAFNESS	OTITIS MEDIA
T8 T9 G41 G44	G41 G3
G20 B62 B63	Si19 T21 Si15 S36
G3 G2	Si3 T5
G41 **Cx9** Liv1	

59. DEAFNESS AND DUMBNESS   *LONG YA*
Section 1

CAUSE OF DISEASE	SYMPTOMS	DIAGNOSTIC FEATURES	MAIN POINTS	SECONDARY POINTS
1. Former Heaven (pre-natal)	Cannot hear or speak.	Deaf and dumb from birth.	Gv20 G2 T17 H5 Gv15	Li4 S36 Si19
2. Latter Heaven (post-natal): prolonged deafness and dumbness resulting from an accident.	As above.	Hearing and speech originally normal; deafness and dumbness occur after illness or accident.	G2 T17 Gv15	T5 H5

Section 2

STUTTERING
Gv4 K5 Cx9

60. SEVERE INFLAMMATION OF THE EYES   *BAO FA HUO YAN*
Section 1

CAUSE OF DISEASE	SYMPTOMS	DIAGNOSTIC FEATURES	MAIN POINTS	SECONDARY POINTS
1. Wind and Heat ascend.	Eye-sockets swollen and painful; eyes shed many tears and are red and itch.	White of the eyes becomes swollen and red; eyes feel rough; photophobia.	G20 B1 Liv2	Li4 G37

Section 2

EYES EASILY BECOME TIRED	CONJUNCTIVITIS
G20 G14 Liv8	T5 Li4 G3
G3 S1 B2 B1	S8 Si3 G20 B10
Cx2 Gv19 B10 Si6	G14 Si18
Gv24a Li4 K1	S44 G15 T3
S8 G16 T23	B1 T23 Liv2 Cx8

PHOTOPHOBIA	BLEPHARITIS
G20 G13 G15	T10 S36 G3
Liv3 B60 Si5	Si4 Li2

STRABISMUS
Circumorbital points

GLAUCOMA
G20 Li1 Si1
K1 B62 S43
G3 Gv24

CRIES TOO EASILY
K5 B15
Cx7 Gv20
S8 G37 Si3

PTERYGION
G14 B2 B1 T23
Or other circumorbital points (A. Chamfrault after
Tsou Lieun)

SPOTS IN FRONT OF EYES
Liv2 Liv14 Li4 Si4
G20 G19 G18
G3 B2

STYE
L11 Si7 B1 (A. Chamfrault)

61. BIRDS EYE (?) *CHIAO MU*

Section 1

CAUSE OF DISEASE	SYMPTOMS	DIAGNOSTIC FEATURES	MAIN POINTS	SECONDARY POINTS
Liver Wind Evil and Fire rush upwards into the eyes.	Eyes dull in the evening, bright in the morning; eyes feel extremely rough and itch.	At night can only see things directly below the eyes, cannot see anything above.	G20 B1 B18	Li4 S36

Section 2

	CATARACT	CATARACT—cont.
	Occasionally effective in very early stage	T1 B1 B67 Gv28
	Li4 L9 Liv3 G1	S6 G41
	G20 B8	B2 G14 S14

62. PURULENT RHINORRHOEA *BI YUAN*

Section 1

CAUSE OF DISEASE	SYMPTOMS	DIAGNOSTIC FEATURES	MAIN POINTS	SECONDARY POINTS
Wind and Heat in brain.	Thick mucus flows incessantly from nose.	Mucus foul-smelling and yellow.	G20 Gv23 Li20	Li4 G40

Section 2

	NASAL CATARRH	SINUSITIS
	Li4 L7	K8 Liv8
	G1 B2 Li20	Gv26 S7 S1 S3 G14 B2 Gv28
	G20 Gv14 Gv16 Gv20 Gv28	B64 S45 S40
	Cx8 Si2	Si1 Si18

NASAL CATARRH
S3 S45
T17 G15 G19

RHINORRHOEA ASSOCIATED WITH
TENSION
Cx6 Cx7
Gv16 Gv12 Gv24a
T5 K10

HAY FEVER
Liv8 K9 Li4
Li19 Gv23 Gv16
B10 B11 B12
Cv17 Cv20

SNEEZING
L5
G4 S8 B12

SINUSITIS
K3 B62
Li11 Li17
Li20 Gv23
B12 G20

ANOSMIA
Sp4 L9
B3 B4 B1
B56 B60
B17 S12
Li20 Li19 Gv25 Gv16 B10

NASAL POLYPS
Li20 Li19
Gv28 Gv26 Gv25 Gv24 Gv14 Gv15 Gv16
K3 L7

63. BREAST ABSCESS *RU YONG*
Section 1

CAUSE OF DISEASE	SYMPTOMS	DIAGNOSTIC FEATURES	MAIN POINTS	SECONDARY POINTS
Liver Qi depressed and congealed; stomach Hot and obstructed.	Breast red, swollen, inflamed and painful; at first alternately hot and cold; swelling hard and painful.	(no observations)	G21 L7 B54	B17 Sp10

Section 2

BREAST ABSCESS
L7 Si1
Sp18 G41
Li8 S34
Cx7 Cv17

64. GOOSE-FOOT WIND (Skin disease of hands only) *E ZHANG FENG*
Section 1

CAUSE OF DISEASE	SYMPTOMS	DIAGNOSTIC FEATURES	MAIN POINTS	SECONDARY POINTS
Blood scorched and affected by Wind which causes it to congeal.	Centre of palm of hand mottled purple and white, changing to white skin; it is hard, thick, dry, withered and cracked; gradually spreads to whole hand.	(no observations)	Cx8	Cx6 Cx7 H8

65. DISEASES OF THE KNEE (Crane-knee Wind) *HAO XI FENG*

Section 1

CAUSE OF DISEASE	SYMPTOMS	DIAGNOSTIC FEATURES	MAIN POINTS	SECONDARY POINTS
1. Affected by Wind and Cold outside; spleen Damp flows downwards.	At first pain inside the patella; after some time it becomes swollen and the thigh becomes increasingly thin.	Colour of swollen skin does not change; Pulse Slowed-down and without strength; tongue pale.	S34 Sp10 Sp9 G34	S36 Sp6
2. Liver and kidney Yin deficient; Damp and Heat flow downwards.	Knee joints red, swollen and painful; Jing Shen does not move; if prolonged the skin and flesh above and below the knee become withered and contracted.	Pulse Fine and Rapid; tongue red, not furred.	S34 Sp9 Sp6	K7 Liv2

Section 2

See No. 35.

66. BERIBERI (Foot Qi) *JIAO QI*

Section 1

CAUSE OF DISEASE	SYMPTOMS	DIAGNOSTIC FEATURES	MAIN POINTS	SECONDARY POINTS
1. Damp: Damp and Heat flow downwards.	Both feet swollen and painful and intensely hot.	Pulse Slippery and Rapid; tongue furred, slippery and greasy.	S28 Sp9 S36	Liv2 G34
2. Dry: affected by Wind and Cold outside.	Alternately hot and cold; both feet painful; no swelling or fever.	Pulse Wiry and Tight; tongue thinly furred white.	T5 Sp9 G34	K7 B60

67. PROLAPSE OF RECTUM *TUO GANG*

Section 1

CAUSE OF DISEASE	SYMPTOMS	DIAGNOSTIC FEATURES	MAIN POINTS	SECONDARY POINTS
1. Qi Empty, sinks downwards.	Prolapse of rectum after defaecation; does not retract.	Pulse Deep and Weak; face white; dyspnoea.	Gv20 Cv8 Gv1	B25 B24 S25 S36
2. Lungs Cold.	Prolapse of rectum, does not retract.	Pulse Empty or Slowed-down; face white; tongue substance pale.	B13 B25 Cv8 Gv1	Cv17 S25 B24 S36

CAUSE OF DISEASE	SYMPTOMS	DIAGNOSTIC FEATURES	MAIN POINTS	SECONDARY POINTS
3. Constant diarrhoea: spleen and stomach Empty and Cold.	Prolapse of rectum after diarrhoea; does not retract.	Pulse Deep and Fine; face yellow; tongue pale; prolapse after each bout of diarrhoea.	Gv20 Cv8 B20 B21 Gv1	B25 S25 S36 Sp6
4. Damp and Heat ascend.	Prolapse of rectum, painful.	Pulse Deep and Slippery; tongue furred yellow and greasy; dysuria, urine red; rectum painful.	Gv20 Gv1 B25	S28 S36 Sp6

Section 2

PROLAPSE OF RECTUM
B58 B57 K5 B62
Gv1 Gv4 Gv20
Sp4 Sp12 S15 S25

PROLAPSE OF RECTUM—cont.
Cx6 T7 T3
B31 B32 B33 B34 B35

Diseases of Women

68. IRREGULAR MENSTRUATION *YUE JING BU TIAO*

Section 1

CAUSE OF DISEASE	SYMPTOMS	DIAGNOSTIC FEATURES	MAIN POINTS	SECONDARY POINTS
1. Blood Hot, Fire brilliant.	Period comes early; large amounts of blood, coloured purple and lumpy; heart troubled and burning; head dizzy; the Five Hearts are troubled and hot.	Pulse Deep and Slippery or Rapid; point of tongue red.	Cv4 Cv3	Cx6 Sp6
2. Blood Hot, Qi Empty.	Period comes early; small amounts of pale blood; dyspnoea; body weary.	Pulse Deep and Slowed-down and without strength; tongue not furred; little saliva.	Cv6 Cv4	Sp10 Sp6
3. Blood Cold and Empty.	Period comes late; small amounts of pale blood; lower abdomen cold and painful.	Pulse Slowed-down and Rough.	Cv4 Cv3 Sp10	S36 Sp6
4. Blood Cold, Qi Empty; both unable to strengthen the lower part of the body.	Period comes late; large amounts of blood which cannot be stopped.	Pulse Deep and Weak.	Gv12 B38 Cv6	Sp10 Sp6
5. Liver and kidney depressed.	Periods irregular, may come early or late.	Pulse Wiry and Rough.	B17 B18 Cv3	Sp8 Sp6

Section 2

IRREGULAR MENSTRUATION
Sp6 Sp10 S25 Cv4 Cv6
Sp4 Cx6
B23

69. DYSMENORRHOEA *TONG JING*

Section 1

CAUSE OF DISEASE	SYMPTOMS	DIAGNOSTIC FEATURES	MAIN POINTS	SECONDARY POINTS
1. Blood Hot, Qi depressed; dead blood blocked and congealed.	Period comes early; lower abdomen painful; blood purple and lumpy.	Pulse Wiry and Rough.	B17 Cv6 Cv4 Liv13	Sp10 Cx6

CAUSE OF DISEASE	SYMPTOMS	DIAGNOSTIC FEATURES	MAIN POINTS	SECONDARY POINTS
2. Qi and blood Empty and deficient; Water does not submerge Wood (Note 1).	Period comes late; lower abdomen painful.	Pulse Slowed-down, Rough and Weak.	Cv6 Cv4	Sp6
3. Blood Empty and Cold.	Lower abdomen painful during period; dragging pain in both sides; limbs and loins aching and tired.	Pulse Deep and Tight.	Cv4 Cv3	S36 Sp6

NOTES

1. *See chapter on The Five Elements in 'Acupuncture'.*

Section 2

DYSMENORRHOEA
Liv8 L7 Sp6 K3
B62 G35 Li4 S28
Liv14 K15

DYSMENORRHOEA—cont.
B31 B32 B33 B34
Gv12

70. AMENORRHOEA   *JING BI*

Section 1

CAUSE OF DISEASE	SYMPTOMS	DIAGNOSTIC FEATURES	MAIN POINTS	SECONDARY POINTS
1. Blood obstructed: caused by Cold Qi lodging in Womb Gate.	Menstruation ceases; lower abdomen swollen and hard; becoming larger daily as though pregnant.	Pulse Deep, Tight and Rough.	Cv4 Cv3 B23	Sp6
2. Blood deficient: Grief injures heart and spleen.	Menstruation ceases; appetite decreases rapidly; skin and flesh dry and emaciated; Shen tired; body lethargic.	Pulse Weak-floating and Fine and without strength.	B38 B20 B21	Cv4 S36
3. Blood withered: bearing and/or suckling large number of children; excessive sexual intercourse; Jing exhausted. (Note 1).	Menstruation ceases; little appetite; skin dry and withered; incessant coughing.	Pulse Deep, Fine and Rapid; cheekbones red after midday; face dry, white and mat.	B37 B38	Cv4 S36

NOTES

1. *It is important to realise that Jing has a wider meaning than 'sperm', and is present in women. It is the fusion of the male and female Jing which creates life. (See also Introduction.)*

AMENORRHOEA
Li4 Sp6
B38 S36 S25
Liv8
Cv3 Cv2 S29
B60 Cv2 Gv1

STERILITY
Sp5 Cv3 (Chamfrault)
K3 L7
S30 K5

71. MENORRHAGIA *BENG LOU*

Section 1

CAUSE OF DISEASE	SYMPTOMS	DIAGNOSTIC FEATURES	MAIN POINTS	SECONDARY POINTS
1. Blood excessively Hot; Heat rushes into and injures the Vessel of Conception.	Slight trickle or sudden heavy flow of blood during periods; blood is dark purple, coagulated and lumpy; abdomen swollen and painful.	Pulse Wiry and Rapid or Hollow; tongue substance red.	K14 Cv3	Sp10 Sp6
2. Mental anxiety injures spleen and causes it to be Empty and unable to obtain blood.	Slight trickle or sudden heavy flow of blood which does not cease; whole body weary and lethargic; desires to lie down; little appetite; palpitation of the heart; loins ache.	Pulse Fine and Weak and without strength; face greenish-yellow; lips white; tongue shiny, no saliva.	B20 Cv6 Liv13	Sp6
3. Violent anger injures liver; liver does not store blood; blood Hot and moves wildly.	Slight trickle or sudden heavy flow of blood which does not cease; chest-ribs swollen and full; limbs and loins ache; throat dry; head dizzy.	Pulse Deep and Wiry; face bluish-yellow; lips at first red then white; tongue shiny and slippery.	Liv13 Cv6 Cv3	Liv1 Sp1

Section 2

MENORRHAGIA
Sp1 Liv3 H5
Cv6 B55 S18
H1 B54 Sp2

72. VAGINAL DISCHARGE *DAI XIA*

Section 1

CAUSE OF DISEASE	SYMPTOMS	DIAGNOSTIC FEATURES	MAIN POINTS	SECONDARY POINTS
1. White discharge: spleen meridian not protected; Damp Evil sinks downwards.	White discharge like saliva or mucus, occurring in middle age; if severe is foul-smelling.	Pulse Slowed-down and Slippery.	B20 G26 B23 Cv3	Sp9 Sp6

CAUSE OF DISEASE	SYMPTOMS	DIAGNOSTIC FEATURES	MAIN POINTS	SECONDARY POINTS
2. Green discharge: liver meridian Damp and Hot.	Discharge like green-bean juice, thick and glutinous; foul-smelling.	Pulse Wiry, Slippery, Weak-floating and Slowed-down.	B18 Liv13 Cv3	Sp6 Liv2
3. Black discharge: Fire very Hot and abundant.	Discharge like black-bean juice; foul-smelling; lower abdomen painful; micturition as though pierced with a knife; vagina swollen; face red.	Pulse Slippery and Rapid or Deep and Rapid.	B23 G26 Cv3	Sp6 K6
4. Yellow discharge: Damp Evil in Vessel of Conception.	Discharge like the thick juice of yellow tea and foul-smelling.	Pulse Wiry, Slowed-down and Weak-floating.	B20 B22 G26 Cv4	Sp6 Sp4
5. Red discharge: Damp and Heat injure the blood.	Discharge red like blood but is not blood; slight continuous discharge.	Pulse Deep and Slippery.	B15 B17 B18 Cv3	Sp10 Sp6

Section 2

VAGINAL DISCHARGE
Sp10 Cv2 Cv3
Gvl Gv2 Gv4
B31 B32 B33 B34

VAGINAL DISCHARGE—cont.
G26 S25 Liv3
Liv11 Sp8 K12

73. FIBROIDS AND ABDOMINAL TUMOURS (Note 1) *ZHENG JIA*

Section 1

CAUSE OF DISEASE	SYMPTOMS	DIAGNOSTIC FEATURES	MAIN POINTS	SECONDARY POINTS
1. Food Zheng: poor food after menstruation or confinement produces cold matter.	Hard lump in abdomen which cannot be moved; increases rapidly in size.	Pulse Deep and Slippery.	Cv12 Liv13 B20 B21	Si4 S36 Sp4 S25 Cv6
2. Blood Zheng: after menstruation or confinement Zang Qi Empty; affected by cold Wind which contests with the blood.	Hard lump in abdomen which cannot be moved; sides and abdomen swollen and painful; interior of body hot; heart troubled.	Pulse Hard.	Cv12 Liv13 B17 B18 B20	G26 S25 Cv4 Sp10 Sp6
3. Jia: cold Wind in-	Jia Qi attacks upwards and down-	Pulse Deep and Tight.	Cv12	B13

CAUSE OF DISEASE	SYMPTOMS	DIAGNOSTIC FEATURES	MAIN POINTS	SECONDARY POINTS
vades the body; Qi and blood congealed and obstructed.	wards causing pain; moves when pressed.		Cv4 B17 B20 B21	Sp10 Liv3 S36 Sp6

NOTES
1. *Jianshi gives Zheng as a hard and immovable swelling in the abdomen; and Jia as movable when pressed and not constantly present—'sometimes scatters sometimes appears'.*

74. PROLAPSE OF VAGINA   *YIN TING*
Section 1

CAUSE OF DISEASE	SYMPTOMS	DIAGNOSTIC FEATURES	MAIN POINTS	SECONDARY POINTS
1. Qi Empty and descends.	Inside of vagina projects like a snake or a mushroom or a cock's-comb. Secondary symptoms: dragging pain; large quantities of clear urine.	Pulse Weak-floating tongue pale.	Cv6 Cv4 Sp6	Liv1 Liv2
2. Damp and Heat flow downwards.	As above. Secondary symptoms: vagina swollen and painful; urine red.	Pulse Rapid; tongue red.	Cv7 S28 Cv3	Sp6 Liv2

Section 2

PROLAPSUS UTERI
K1 Liv1
H8 K3 Liv8
B31 B32

75. PRURITIS VULVAE   *YIN YANG*
Section 1

CAUSE OF DISEASE	SYMPTOMS	DIAGNOSTIC FEATURES	MAIN POINTS	SECONDARY POINTS
Damp and Heat produce Worms, (see Notes to No. 55 Tooth-ache).	Lower part of vagina itches; slight incontinence of urine.	Pulse Wiry and Slowed-down; tongue furred, slippery and greasy.	Cv3 Sp10 Sp6	B54 Liv2

Section 2

PRURITIS VULVAE
S31 S30 Liv11
Cv3 Gv1 Cv1
H8 K10 B60

76. UNPLEASANT SYMPTOMS DURING PREGNANCY *REN ZHEN WU ZU*

Section 1

CAUSE OF DISEASE	SYMPTOMS	DIAGNOSTIC FEATURES	MAIN POINTS	SECONDARY POINTS
1. Spleen and stomach Empty and Weak; Phlegm-fluid stored inside the body.	Vomiting phlegm; heart troubled; head dizzy; limbs tired and lethargic; likes sour foods and dislikes normal food.	Pulse Slippery and without strength or Slowed-down; tongue lightly furred white.	B20 B21 Cx6 Cv12 Liv13 (last 2 only up to 5th month).	Liv2 S36 Sp4
2. Liver Qi depressed and congealed; Qi does not circulate.	Chest-ribs swollen and full; head and eyes dizzy; hates cold, likes heat; chest perturbed; likes sour foods and is particular in choice of food; may be unable to eat; body tired and has no strength; mouth may be dry; may be constipated.	Pulse Deep and Slippery and without strength; both Connecting Pulses Empty and Wiry; tongue furred white.	B18 Liv13 B20 B21	Liv2 S43 Cx6 S36
3. Liver rebels; stomach Hot.	Nausea and vomiting; heart troubled, anxious and annoyed; likes the cold and to drink cool fluids; dislikes food; vomitus sour; head painful; dislikes the heat; constipated; urine red.	Pulse Wiry, Slippery and Rapid; tongue lightly furred yellow.	B18 B19 B21 S36 Cx6	Liv3 S44 G34

Section 2

NAUSEA AND VOMITING OF PREGNANCY
Liv8 G40 S45
Cx6 Sp6 L5 L9

77. ECLAMPSIA (Note 1) *ZI XIAN*

Section 1

CAUSE OF DISEASE	SYMPTOMS	DIAGNOSTIC FEATURES	MAIN POINTS	SECONDARY POINTS
Caused by heart and liver meridians being depressed and Hot.	Sudden collapse in pregnant women; cramp and muscular spasms; becomes unconscious; normal when conscious.	Pulse Wiry and Slippery or Stopped.	Gv26 G20 Gv16 B10	S36 Cx6 G34

NOTES

1. *The Chinese heading is 'Child' plus Xian, one of the three subdivisions of No. 26 Convulsions.*

ECLAMPSIA
K2 Cx7
G21 G34
Si14 S36

78. PROLONGED LABOUR   *ZHI CHAN*

Section 1

CAUSE OF DISEASE	SYMPTOMS	DIAGNOSTIC FEATURES	MAIN POINTS	SECONDARY POINTS
Liking for leisure, no physical work, excessive sleeping and resting cause Qi and blood to become obstructed.	Full-term foetus is not born.	Despite labour pains foetus does not turn and move; Pulse Slowed-down.	Li4 Sp6	G21 B67

Section 2

PROLONGED LABOUR
L14 S30 Sp15
Sp6 B67 Gv2
B23 B33

79. RETAINED PLACENTA   *TAI YI BU XIA*

Section 1

CAUSE OF DISEASE	SYMPTOMS	DIAGNOSTIC FEATURES	MAIN POINTS	SECONDARY POINTS
Excessive and prolonged physical toil; Qi weak, blood congealed.	Placenta does not descend; abdomen swollen and painful.	Pulse Empty; face hoary-white; tongue purple.	G21 Cv3 B60	Li4 Sp6

Section 2

RETAINED PLACENTA
G21 Sp6
K3 B67 B47 B32
Cv3 Cv5 Cv6 Cv7

80. POST-NATAL SPASMS   *CHAN HOU JING LÜAN*

Section 1

CAUSE OF DISEASE	SYMPTOMS	DIAGNOSTIC FEATURES	MAIN POINTS	SECONDARY POINTS
1. Blood deficient after	Muscular spasms and pain; unable	Pulse Floating and Slowed-	Cx3	Li11

CAUSE OF DISEASE	SYMPTOMS	DIAGNOSTIC FEATURES	MAIN POINTS	SECONDARY POINTS
confinement; Wind Evil ascends and invades the body.	to stretch; no sweating.	down; tongue lightly furred white.	T5	Li4
2. Blood deficient after confinement; unable to use muscles.	Muscular spasms and pain; sweating.	Pulse Empty; tongue pale	Cx3 Si3	Cv6

81. PAIN IN LOWER ABDOMEN AFTER CONFINEMENT
CHAN HOU SHAO FU TONG

Section 1

CAUSE OF DISEASE	SYMPTOMS	DIAGNOSTIC FEATURES	MAIN POINTS	SECONDARY POINTS
1. Dead blood has not been cleansed.	Slight pain in lower abdomen.	Pulse Rough.	S25 Cv4	Sp10 Sp6
2. Water stored up in lower part of body.	Lower abdomen hard and painful; dysuria with slight urinary incontinence; abdomen swollen and painful.	Micturition rough; urinary incontinence; Pulse Deep; tongue furred and slippery.	Cv3 S28	Sp9 K7
3. Dead blood.	Lower abdomen hard, resists pressure; polyuria.	Polyuria; tongue dark purple; Pulse Rough and Blocked.	S25 Cv4 K14	Sp10 Sp6

Section 2

PAIN IN LOWER ABDOMEN
AFTER CONFINEMENT
Sp6 Cv6

POST PARTUM VAGINAL DISCHARGE
Liv6 Sp6
Cv6 Cv3 Cv2
T7

PUERPERAL FEVER
B25 B31
Li10 S36 Li4 Sp6

82. INSUFFICIENT LACTATION   RU SHAO

Section 1

CAUSE OF DISEASE	SYMPTOMS	DIAGNOSTIC FEATURES	MAIN POINTS	SECONDARY POINTS
1. Blood Empty; excessive bleeding during confinement.	Small amount of milk in breast; face very white.	Eats little; Pulse Empty; tongue pale.	Cv17 (moxa) Si1	Li4 S36 Sp6

CAUSE OF DISEASE	SYMPTOMS	DIAGNOSTIC FEATURES	MAIN POINTS	SECONDARY POINTS
2. Qi Mai blocked and Cold.	Small amount of milk in breast; heart troubled; agitated and impetuous.	Pulse Large; tongue red.	Cv17 (moxa) Si1 G21	L7

Section 2

INSUFFICIENT LACTATION
Si1 H1 Cv17 S18
B38 (S. de Morant)
G41 Cv3

Diseases of Children

83. ACUTE CONVULSIONS *JI JING FENG*

Section 1

CAUSE OF DISEASE	SYMPTOMS	DIAGNOSTIC FEATURES	MAIN POINTS	SECONDARY POINTS
1. Heart meridian Hot; eyes see strange things, ears hear strange noises.	Convulsions; easily startled; frequent weeping at night.	Pulse Overflowing and Rapid; face blue-green; tongue red.	Gv14 Gv26	Si4 K1
2. Heart and liver Fire abundant; affected by Wind and Cold from outside.	Body hot but no sweating; convulsions; constipation.	Pulse Floating and Overflowing, Slippery and Rapid; tongue furred yellowish-white.	Gv13 Si4 Liv3	Li4 L7
3. Phlegm abundant, produces Wind.	Phlegm bubbling; breathing hurried; mouth tightly closed; spasms of limbs.	Pulse Slippery.	Gv12 Cv12	L11 T1
4. Upper Warmer Hot and abundant.	Body hot; heart troubled and anxious; spasms of limbs; face and lips blue-green; small quantities of red urine; mouth parched.	Pulse Overflowing and Rapid.	Gv26 K1	L11 T1

Section 2

SCREAMING FITS	PETIT MAL
K5 L9	B62

84. MILD CONVULSIONS *MAN JING FENG*

Section 1

CAUSE OF DISEASE	SYMPTOMS	DIAGNOSTIC FEATURES	MAIN POINTS	SECONDARY POINTS
1. Constitution previously weak; spleen Empty; liver abundant and containing Phlegm.	Mild intermittent convulsions; face blue-green and white; body not hot; much phlegm.	Pulse Slowed-down, Minute and Slippery and without strength.	Gv14 Gv12	Cv4 S36

154

CAUSE OF DISEASE	SYMPTOMS	DIAGNOSTIC FEATURES	MAIN POINTS	SECONDARY POINTS
2. Caused by having previously taken Cold Medicine as cure for severe convulsions (see No. 83).	Very mild spasms; eyes slightly open when asleep; not of excitable nature; stools blue-green.	Pulse Empty and Slow; urine blue-green and white.	Gv12 Cv6	G34

Section 2

AFRAID OF DARK
K10 Gv20 Cx9

85. CHRONIC SPLEEN WIND (?)   *MAN PI FENG*

Section 1

CAUSE OF DISEASE	SYMPTOMS	DIAGNOSTIC FEATURES	MAIN POINTS	SECONDARY POINTS
1. Continuous diarrhoea and vomiting all day long; spleen Yang badly injured.	Closes eyes and shakes head; face dark; sweat appears on forehead; troubled sleep; limbs cold.	Pulse Deep and Slow and without strength.	Gv20 Gv12 B20	Sp4
2. Extremely ill all day long; spleen Empty and does not move; muscles are not nourished by the blood; Emptiness produces Wind.	Troubled sleep with eyes partly open; limbs cold; face dull and colourless; spasms almost imperceptible.	Pulse Weak and without strength.	Gv12 B20 Cv6	Liv3

86. PARALYSIS IN CHILDREN, INCLUDING POLIOMYELITIS   *XIAO ER WEI BI*

Section 1

CAUSE OF DISEASE	SYMPTOMS	DIAGNOSTIC FEATURES	MAIN POINTS	SECONDARY POINTS
1. Wei: lungs Hot, bronchi Dry.	Both legs paralysed and weak; unable to walk.	Legs weak and soft to touch; face white.	press points on spine with bamboo needle G20 B11 G34	Li4 T4 Si4 G30 K8 K3 B62

CAUSE OF DISEASE	SYMPTOMS	DIAGNOSTIC FEATURES	MAIN POINTS	SECONDARY POINTS
2. Bi: the combined Evils of Wind, Cold and Damp.	Both legs stiff and straight; walking difficult.	Legs stiff and hard when pressed; face blue-green.	Gv12 G20 G30	G34 Sp9

Section 2   See Nos. 35, 37.

87. COUGHING   *KE SOU*

Section 1

CAUSE OF DISEASE	SYMPTOMS	DIAGNOSTIC FEATURES	MAIN POINTS	SECONDARY POINTS
1. Wind and Cold cough: Wind and Cold enter lungs.	Sputum clear and white; coughing; dislikes the cold; nose blocked.	Pulse Floating; tongue lightly furred white.	B12 B13 Cv6	Li4 L7
2. Hot lungs cough: Hot Phlegm in lungs.	Face red; throat dry; sputum yellow and glutinous; coughing.	Pulse Rapid; tongue thickly furred white and fairly dry.	B12 B13	L5 L10
3. Accumulated food cough: accumulation of food produces Phlegm; Heat rebels against the lungs.	Breathing hurried; sputum obstructed; coughing; bad smell of food may remain in mouth; stools foul-smelling.	Pulse Slippery; tongue lightly furred yellow.	B13 B20 B21	L6 Cv12 S36
4. Wind and Heat cough: Wind enters lungs, changes to Heat and causes Phlegm	Face and lips red; mucus from nose concentrated; does not dislike the cold; coughing; sputum slightly concentrated.	Pulse Floating and Rapid.	B12 B13	L5 L9
5. Full Fire cough: Full Fire in lungs; Phlegm thick and turbid.	Face red during coughing bouts; violent vomiting with much noise; sputum concentrated; mouth parched.	Pulse Overflowing and Full; tongue yellow and dry.	Cv22 Cv17 (moxa)	L6 L10
6. Empty lung cough: Wind enters lungs, changes to Heat and is not cured for a long time.	Protracted cough with weak breathing; sweating during coughing bouts; voice low; dyspnoea.	Right Inch Pulse Weak-floating.	B13 Gv12 B38	Cv6 S36
7. Damp and drinking cough: excessive drinking of tea or water may injure the body and produce cold.	Face yellowish-white; large amounts of thin, non-glutinous sputum; stools watery; chest melancholy.	Tongue furred white and greasy; Pulse Slowed-down.	B13 B21	S36 L6

88. INDIGESTION   *SHANG SHI*

Section 1

CAUSE OF DISEASE	SYMPTOMS	DIAGNOSTIC FEATURES	MAIN POINTS	SECONDARY POINTS
Food and drink injure the spleen. The Classic (Nei Jing?) says: 'If food and drink rebel of their own accord, the intestines and stomach are injured.'	Fever; dislikes food; belches sour breath; dislikes the smell of food; desires to vomit but cannot; dyspnoea; indigestion; swallows sour saliva; abdomen painful and swollen.	Stools sour and foul-smelling; hot at night, cool in morning; feet cold; stomach hot; Pulse Full and has strength.	Cv12 Liv13 B20 B21	Cx6 Sp4 Cv21 S36

89. BLOCKAGE DISEASES   *PI JI*

Section 1

CAUSE OF DISEASE	SYMPTOMS	DIAGNOSTIC FEATURES	MAIN POINTS	SECONDARY POINTS
Eating and drinking irregular; intestines and stomach completely full; semi-digested food obstructed and so over-flows; also affected by Cold Qi which congeals.	Hard lump like overturned cup below left ribs; at first like chicken's egg, gradually increasing in size; heavy sweating; emaciated; likes to drink cold water.	Pulse Hard.	XB2 (moxa) Liv13	Sp3

90. *GAN JI* (see Note 1)

Section 1

CAUSE OF DISEASE	SYMPTOMS	DIAGNOSTIC FEATURES	MAIN POINTS	SECONDARY POINTS
1. Spleen Gan: milk and food not properly regulated, forming a blockage and generating Heat which wastes and destroys blood and Qi; Gan Heat injures the spleen.	Face yellow; flesh wasted away; body hot and lethargic; region below heart blocked and full; stomach and abdomen hard; likes to eat mud (?); head large, neck fine; occasional diarrhoea and vomiting; stools smell rotten and are glutinous.	Right Connecting Pulse Deep, Fine and Rapid; face yellow.	XA2 (let yellow fluid.)	S36 Sp4

CAUSE OF DISEASE	SYMPTOMS	DIAGNOSTIC FEATURES	MAIN POINTS	SECONDARY POINTS
2. Liver Gan: unlimited food and drink; accumulated Heat becomes Gan; Gan Heat injures the liver.	Face, eyes and fingernails blue-green; eyes diseased and watery; shakes head and rubs eyes; thick fluid flows from ears; large blue-green veins on abdomen; emaciated; thirsty; stools blue-green.	Right Connecting Pulse Wiry and Rapid; face blue-green.	as above	S36 Liv2
3. Heart Gan: food and drink obstructed; accumulated Heat becomes Gan; stored up Heat rises into heart.	Face and eyes red; high fever; sweating; continuously agitated; snaps teeth and moves tongue; mouth and tongue dry and burning; thirsty; sores in mouth; chest-diaphragm full and melancholy; body emaciated.	Pulse Overflowing and Rapid; face red.	as above	S36 H8
4. Lung Gan: food and drink not properly regulated; accumulated Heat becomes Gan; stored up Heat rises to lungs.	Face white; coughing; hair becomes dry and withered; flesh and skin dry and burning; high fever; usually emits blue-green pus from nose; sores develop in nostrils.	Right Inch Pulse Slippery and Rapid.	as above	S36 L10
5. Kidney Gan: food and drink not properly regulated; accumulated Heat becomes Gan; Gan Heat injures kidney.	Face very dark; bleeding from gums; breath foul-smelling; feet very cold; abdomen painful; diarrhoea; associated with incomplete knitting together of fontanel, or late teething and walking.	Pulse Fine and Rapid.	as above	S36 K2
6. Innocent Gan: food and drink not properly regulated; accumulated Heat becomes Gan; Gan Heat becomes Poison.	Sores on neck or hard lump inside back of neck; incessant rectal bleeding with pus; body emaciated; face yellow; fever.	Pulse Wiry and Rapid; tongue deep red.	(press points on spine with bamboo needle)	G40 Liv5

NOTES

1. *Gan seems to be a general term for a large number of complaints common in children below the age of 15. Note that whatever the symptoms, food and drink are the cause in each case. The Chinese word Ji in the heading Gan Ji means 'to accumulate' (cf. No. 21 Qi Accumulation Diseases).*

91. VOMITING   *OU TU*

Section 1

CAUSE OF DISEASE	SYMPTOMS	DIAGNOSTIC FEATURES	MAIN POINTS	SECONDARY POINTS
1. Milk injury vomiting: child takes excess of milk which is stopped in the stomach.	Vomits milk; body hot; face yellow; skin puffy.	Pulse Slippery and Rapid.	Cv12 S36	Cx6 Cv21
2. Food injury vomiting: food and drink not properly regulated; excess of greasy foods; obstruction formed in digestive tract.	Stomach and abdomen swollen and hot; mouth foul-smelling; vomitus sour and glutinous; fever.	Pulse Deep and Floating.	Cv12 Liv13 S36	Cv21 Cx6
3. Cold vomiting: excess of food produces cold.	Food eaten in morning vomited in evening; vomitus neither foul-smelling or sour; limbs cold.	Pulse Deep and Slow; face and lips white.	Gv12 B20 B21	S36
4. Hot vomiting: excess of hot, greasy food; Heat accumulates in middle of body.	Food vomited on entering stomach; mouth parched; body hot; lips red; urine red; vomitus sour and watery.	Pulse Rapid.	Cx6 S36	Sp4 S44
5. Empty vomiting: stomach Qi Empty and weak; cannot digest milk and food.	Jing Shen weary and lethargic; continuous vomiting; micturition and defaecation normal; no thirst; eyes open when asleep.	Pulse Empty and Slow.	Gv12 Cv4 B20 B21	S36
6. Full vomiting: milk and food obstructed; stomach Heat attacks upwards.	Chest and abdomen swollen and painful; hard and painful lump in stomach; micturition and defaecation difficult and rough; thirsty, likes cool fluids; vomitus sour and foul-smelling.	Pulse Deep and Full.	S36	T6 Sp4

Section 2

INTERMITTENT ABDOMINAL PAIN
Liv8

Glossary

A short list of translated terms, with their Chinese equivalents, and brief notes on their meaning.

1. Terms used chiefly in the description of symptoms:

ACCUMULATES, ACCUMULATION: *ji* — See Notes to No. 21 Qi-Accumulation Diseases.

CONGEAL: *ning, jie* — Note that as a pulse quality *jie* is translated 'knotted'.

DENSE: *mi* — Generally refers to stools; close-packed, heavy etc.

DEPRESSED: *yu* — May refer to an organ or to one of the functional substances.

DISTRESSED: *fanmen* — Generally refers to heart; a combination of *fan* meaning 'troubled' and *men* meaning 'melancholy'.

HARSH: *cu* — Coarse, rough etc. Generally refers to breathing.

MELANCHOLY: *men* — Refers to chest, heart, abdomen etc.

OBSTRUCT, OBSTRUCTION: *pi, sai, zhi, zu* — No meaningful distinction can be drawn between these four words. Note however that as a pulse quality *zhi* is translated 'blocked'.

THICK: *chou* — Similar to 'dense'; refers to stools or urine.

TROUBLED: *fan* — Refers most frequently to the heart.

2. Other terms:

ANIMAL SOUL: *po* — That aspect of Shen which is controlled by the lungs; see Introduction, part I.

CHEST-DIAPHRAGM: *xiong ge* — Refers to the inside of the chest above the diaphragm.

CHEST-RIBS: *xiong xie* — Refers to the outside of the chest, the ribs. Both terms

CHONG MO:		are commonly used in describing the location of pain etc. One of the Eight Extra Meridians, also known as *xue hai*, the Sea of Blood. Traditionally considered as the centre of all blood in the meridians. See 'Acupuncture', chapter X.
COOL MEDICINE:	*liang yao*	One of the categories of Chinese pharmacology.
DORMANT EVIL:	*fu xie*	See Introduction part II.
DORMANT QI:	*fu qi*	,, ,, ,, ,,
EMPTY:	*xu*	Has two meanings; 'hollow' and 'weak', of which the second is the more common.
EXHAUSTED, EXHAUSTION:	*lao*	A whole group of diseases is associated with *lao*; cf. No. 4 in list of Causes of Disease, Introduction part II.
FIRE OF THE FIVE DESIRES:	*wu zhi zhi huo*	The Five Desires (wu zhi) are the same as the Seven Emotions without Mental anxiety and Alarm. The Fire is the motive force of the emotions.
FIVE EXHAUSTIONS:	*wu lao*	May refer to: (a) the Five Zang organs; (b) Qi, Blood, bone (gu), flesh (rou) and sinew or muscle (jin).
FULL:	*man*	Most commonly used to describe the state of a particular region of the body, e.g. stomach, abdomen etc.
	shi	Describes the condition of the functional substances of the body, e.g. Qi, Blood, Ying, Wei etc. Also a pulse quality.
GREAT POISON:	*da du*	Large amounts of toxic substances in the body; may also indicate a highly toxic variety of Chinese medicines.
JING ENERGY:	*jing li*	The 'external manifestation' is very similar to 'libido' but see Introduction, part I, under Jing.
LOWER ABDOMEN:	*shao fu*	Defined by the Chinese as the region of the body from the navel downwards.

LOWER WARMER:	*xia jiao*	The region of the body between the navel and the small-intestine, principally the liver and kidney. The lower Triple Warmer.
MIDDLE QI:	*zhong qi*	Qi in the organs of the middle of the body, i.e. stomach and spleen. Also known as Middle Warmer Qi. Qi of the middle Triple Warmer.
MIDDLE WARMER:	*zhong jiao*	The region of the body between diaphragm and navel, principally the stomach and spleen. The middle Triple Warmer.
MINISTER FIRE:	*xiang huo*	The Fire in the kidneys; cf. Sovereign Fire.
PHLEGM:	*tan*	Translated as Phlegm only when it occurs as a 'metaphysical' concept (generally in the first column of the translation) or when the alternative, 'sputum', in unsuitable.
PHLEGM-FLUID	*tan yin*	See Notes to No. 6 Gastritis.
QI DOES NOT TRANSFORM:	*qi bu hua*	The numerous variations on these lines are essentially
QI DOES NOT MOVE:	*qi bu dong*	the same process. The Qi may be that of a particular
QI DOES NOT ACTIVATE:	*qi bu xing*	organ, and it may fail to act upon another functional substance, e.g. water, blood, etc. See Introduction, part I under Qi.
SEASONAL EVIL:	*shi xie*	The particular Evil, or Qi, appropriate to the time of year. See Introduction, part II.

SEVEN EMOTIONS: *qi qing* The emotions are:

xi	Joy (Fire)	bei	Sorrow (Metal)
nu	Anger (Wood)	kong	Fear (Water)
you	Obession (Earth)	jing	Alarm
si	Mental Anxiety		

Abnormality of these emotions cause disease; conversely abnormality may result from a disease. See 'Acupuncture', chapter IX.

SEVEN INJURIES:	*qi shang*	Several explanations exist; the most common are:

(a) Excessive eating injures the spleen, Great anger injures the liver.

Lifting heavy weights or sitting on damp ground injures the kidneys.

Drinking cold liquids injures the lungs.

Dark thoughts injure the heart.

Wind, rain, cold and heat injure the Form (xing).

Uncontrolled fear injures Desire (zhi)

See 'Acupuncture' chapter IX.

(b) Extreme fear injures Jing.

Worry and anxiety injure Shen.

Excessive joy injures the Animal Soul (po)

Sadness moving inside injures the Spiritual Soul (hun).

Unrestrained melancholy injures Yi (Mind)

Unrestrained rage injures Zhi (Desire).

Excessive weariness injures Qi.

See Introduction, part I.

SOVEREIGN FIRE:	*jun huo*	The Fire in the kidneys; cf. Minister Fire.
SPIRITUAL SOUL:	*hun*	That aspect of Shen controlled by the liver; cf. Animal Soul.
TRUE YIN:	*zhen yin*	Also called True Water (zhen shui); it is the Fluid in the kidneys. See Introduction, part I.
UPPER WARMER:	*shang jiao*	The part of the body above the diaphragm, principally the heart and lungs. Upper Triple Warmer.
WARM POISON:	*wen du*	(a) Extreme Heat changing to Fire and causing diseases characterised by a rash. (b) One group of the eighth of the causes of disease; see Introduction, part II. One of the chief conditions caused by Warm Poison is mumps.
WEI YANG:		See Wei in Introduction, part I.

WORMS: *chong* The word *chong* embraces insects, reptiles etc. It is one of the nine causes of disease, and may well be the ancient Chinese equivalent of bacteria.

Acupuncture: A New Compilation

(*ZHENJIU XIN BIAN*)

COMPILED BY: YE SIU-TING
PUBLISHED BY: DA XIN PUBLISHING HOUSE, TAIWAN, 1965
Translated by: Frank Liu and Felix Mann

On the whole, I think the sections 'Acupuncture: A New Compilation' and 'Periosteal Acupuncture', are where appropriate, the methods to try first when treating a patient. 'A General Survey of Common Diseases and their Treatment by Acupuncture' (called Section 1 on pages 87 to 164), is also good but less clear due to its traditional classification, and is often therefore only second choice.
'Acupuncture Points used in the Treatment of Specific Diseases or Symptoms' (called Section 2 on pages 87 to 164), is generally not as efficacious as the other three sections.

Strengthening

Tonify CNS. Gv23 Gv22 Gv20 B7 B6 Gv19 Gv16 Gv15 G20 B10 G12
Tonify nose. Gv23 B7
Tonify throat. G20 B10 G21
Tonify lungs and bronchi. Gv12 B13 B37 B38 B16
Prevent influenza. B12 Gv12
Tonify heart. B14 B15 B16 Sp17
Tonify circulation. Cv4 Cv6
Tonify lymphatic circulation. B17 Liv13
Tonify stomach and intestines. B18 B20 B21 B25 B31 S36 S37
Tonify genito-urinary system. Gv4 B23 Gv3 B26 B27 B28 B31/4 Cv4 S28 K13
Tonify endocrine, gonads. Gv20 Gv4 Gv3 Cv4
Tonify muscles. Gv20 Gv13 B11 Gv3 B31
Tonify eye and ear. B18 B23 Gv4 Cv4
Generally tonify body. Cv4 S36 Used for immunization as it strengthens and increases amount of blood.

Sedating

Inflammation of head or five senses. Si3 Li4 G41 B67
Inflammation of mouth and throat. L11 L10 S44 K3
Heart and lung inflammation. P6 P7 L7 L9
Chest inflammation. H8 P6 G34 G40
Stomach and intestine inflammation. S36 Sp4 P6 Liv2
Liver and gall bladder inflammation. G40 Liv3 T5 Li4
Urinary tract inflammation. L7 K3 Liv8 Sp9
General body auto inflammation. B54 L5 10 commandments of fingers and toes
Generally for inflammation use distant points

Eructations. Cv22 Cv12 Cv6 L9 P6 S36 Sp4 Liv1 Sp6
Pain and spasms. Same points as for inflammation
Chronic pain and spasms. Use local points and add points as above
Needling: Acute—strong for short period. Chronic—light for long period

Regulating
Constipation. B25 S25 S28 T6 B57
Increase diuresis. Cv3 Sp9 S36 Sp6
Increase perspiration. Gv14 Li4 T5 L8

General Points
Non-tuberculous lymphatic gland swelling. B18 G21
Non-venereal groin and abdominal lymphatic swelling. B57
Spleen swelling. B44 B46 B20
Pulmonary T.B. Gv12 B13 B16
Heart disease. B15 H7 H5 P6
Kidney disease. B22 B23
Bladder. B33 B28 Cv3
Anus. Gv1 P4 B57 Gv20
Stomach. Cv12 P6 S36 B21
Large intestine. B25 S25 S37
Small intestine. Cv6 B26 B27
Uterus. S28 Cv3 Sp6
Eye. G20 XH3 B1 B2 B18
Nose. Gv23 Li20 Li4
Ear. T17 Si19
Mouth. P7 P9
Toothache. S7 Li4
Throat. L11 L10
Arm. Gv13 B11 Li15 Li11
Leg. G33 G30 B54 G34

Mental. Cv15 Cv13 H7 S40
Malaria. Gv14/13
Jaundice. Gv9 Si4

Acute Inflammation of Throat including symptoms such as aphonia,
soreness, cough, headache.
G20 T2 L10
May add B13 Li10 L11
If due to influenza add Gv16 T5 Li4

Chronic Inflammation of Throat
B10 Si14 G21 Cv22 B13 T2 L10
or G20 Si15 Li17 T17 B12 K7 K3

Tuberculosis of Throat
B10 Gv12 B16
May add B13 Cv22 L5 L9 S36 Sp6
or B14 T17 Li17 L10 T2 S40 Sp10
With fever Gv13 P5
Spontaneous perspiration H6 Si3
Anorexia B20 Cv12 S36

Aphonia
G20 S10 B12 T17 Li4 L10
or B10 Li17 G21 Si13 B13 K3 Liv2

Laryngeal Spasm, mainly in male children under 3
Cv12 Cv6 S36 L11 P9 Li4 Sp1 B67

Tracheitis
B11 B13 Cv22 L5 T5 L8 Sp6

Acute Bronchitis
G20 B10 B12 T5 L8
If after treatment headache remains B12 B13 L5 Li4 T5
If after treatment severe cough or tickle in throat remains Cv22 Sp6

Chronic Bronchitis
B13 Cv22 Cv12 K27 L5 S36
or B12 B10 G21 L9 Cv6 S40
Moxa B10 B13 Gv10 Cv22 Cv17 B20 Cv12 S36 S40

Bronchiectasis
B13 B16 B20 S40 Cv12 Cv6 S36

Bronchial Asthma
B13 B16 Cv22 Cv17 G21 Cv12 Cv6 L7 S36 Sp6
Moxa after initial improvement by needles as above B13 B16 Gv12 Gv10 Cv6 S36

Bronchopneumonia Primary treatment by antibiotics. Acupuncture only of secondary importance.
G20 B11 Gv12 B13 B17 Li11 Li4 S36 S44 T5 Si3 S40 Liv2

Lobar Pneumonia Antibiotics are primary treatment..Acupuncture is only supportive.
With headache and fever G20 B12 B13 Li11 T5 Li4 B60 S44 Liv2
With fever and thirst Gv14 Gv12 B12 B13 B17 Li11 T5 Li4 Li1 K7 H9 S44 Liv2
With cough and pain in chest L5 L9 Li4 Cv12 Liv13 S36 G34 Sp6

Emphysema

B13 B15 B37 L5 Cv12 S36 Sp6
or B12 B16 B38 Li11 Cv6 S40 L9
Moxa B13 B37 B16 B38 B23 G33

Tuberculosis Drug treatment primary, acupuncture secondary.
Use only 5 acupuncture points, as patients are often weak.
With fever Gv14 Gv12 B14 P5 K7
High fever add Li11 Li5 Li4 Sp6 Liv2 S44
Cough B13 B16 B38 L5 L9
Unproductive cough add Cv22 Sp6
Pain due to cough K27 L1 Cv17 Cv13 Cv11 Cv6 S36
Productive cough B20 Cv12 S40
Spontaneous sweating H6 Si3 May add Sp6 K7
Haemoptysis L5 L7 If severe add B17 Li1 Liv2
Diarrhoea B25 S25 Cv6 S37
Headache, backache, pain in throat. Treat local symptoms.
Anorexia Cv12 S36
When patient is better use Moxa B13 B16 Gv12 Cv4 S36

Pleurisy

Headache and fever G20 B12 Gv13 L5 T5 Li4 G34
Dry pleurisy Gv12 B12 any tender points over ribs L5 L9 G34 G41
Wet pleurisy. Same as dry pleurisy but add B13 B15 B16 B18 Sp9 Sp6
If temperature down but chest still painful—chronic type Gv14 Gv13 Gv10
Gv9 B18 Cv9 G34 Liv13 Sp6

Hydrothorax

B13 B15 B18 B23 B25 B27 Cv6 Sp9 Sp6
Use thin needle on vertebrae T4 to L4 and ribs below T6

Angina Pectoris

G20 B11 G21 B15 B18 L4 L5 P6

If patient has an attack of angina pectoris during treatment use L4 L6 P6

Acute Endocarditis

L4 Li11 P6 H7 Sp6 K1 Liv3 S42

Valvular Disease

G20 G21 B11 B15 Cv12 Cv6

or B10 B12 B28 B16 Cv11 Cv4

For oedema B23 B32 S36 Sp6 B22 B27 Sp9 K7

Acute Myocarditis

B11 B12 Gv12 B13 Si8 P7

Fatty Heart

G20 G21 B11 B15 Cv12 Cv6 T5 S36

or B10 B12 B38 B16 Cv11 Cv4 S37

Palpitations

G20 G21 B12 B15 P7 S36

or B10 B11 B14 B16 P6 Cv12 Cv6 Sp6

Arteriosclerosis (Liver Yang)

G20 G21 B38 B15 B23 S25 S28 Li15 Li10 G31 S36 Sp6 B60 S41

Shoulder Pain

G20 B11 Si14 Si13 Li15 Li11 Local painful points

Anaemia
B17 B20 B22 B25 Cv4 S36
With tinnitus Si19 T17
With vertigo, headache G20 XH3 S8 T23
With palpitations B15 Cv11
With nausea and vomiting Cv13 Cv12

Chlorosis-Anaemia
Gv20 B10 Gv12 Gv9 B20 B22 Cv4 S36 Sp6

Leukaemia
B20 B18 B17 B22 Gv4 Cv4 S36

DIGESTIVE DISEASES

Mouth Ulcers and Monilia
XM2 Cv23 S6 S4 Li10 Li4 P7 S44
With fever G20 Gv12 Li11

Aphthous Stomatitis
G20 B10 Gv12 Cv24 Cv23 S4 Li11 Li4 T2

Tonsillitis
Acute G20 B10 B11 L5 L11 Li1
Chronic B10 B11 L10 T2

Mumps
G20 B11 Li11 B10 T5 Li4 T2

Sialorrhea
G20 B10 S6 S4 Cv23

Toothache
S7 Li4
Supplementary points G20 B12

Acute Pharyngitis
G20 B10 B11 Li10 Li4 L11 Li1 K3

Chronic Pharyngitis
B10 B11 Gv12 B17 B18 Li17 Cv23 T2 L10

Oesophagitis
B11 B12 Si15 Gv12 G21 Cv22 Cv17 Cv13 Li10 S36 P6 S44

Stricture of Oesophagus
B11 G21 B14 B17 Cv22 Cv17 Cv13 P6 Li10 S36 S40

Spasm of Oesophagus
G20 B11 B13 Cv17 Cv13 Cv6 Cv3 P3 S36 Sp6
or B10 G21 B14 Cv18 Cv14 Cv4 P6 Sp8

Paralysis of Oesophagus
G20 B10 Si15 G21 B13 B15 B18

Acute Gastritis
B17 B19 B21 Cv22 Cv12 Li10 P6 S36 Sp4

Chronic Gastritis
B18 B21 Cv13 Cv11 S19 S21 P6 S36
or B20 B22 Cv12 S20 S23 S37 Sp4

Gastric Spasm
B18 B20 B22 Cv12 Cv6 S36 S44
or B19 B21 B23 Cv11 S37 Liv2

Dilation of Stomach
B18 B20 B22 Cv14 Cv12 S19 S21 S36
or B19 B21 Cv13 S20 Cv11 S37

Gastric Ulcer
G20 B11 B17 B19 B20 S36
or B10 G21 B18 B21 B22 S37

Gastroptosis
B10 B11 B17 B18 B20 B22 S20 S21

Nervous Dyspepsia
B10 B17 B20 B22 Cv13 Cv11 Cv6 S36
or B11 B18 B21 B44 Cv14 Cv12 S37

Neurogenic Vomiting
G20 B10 B21 K21 Cv12 P3 Cv11 S44 Liv3

Gastric Hyperacidity
B10 B11 B17 B18 B20 Cv12 S25 S36

Atony of Stomach
B18 B20 B22 Cv13 Cv12 Cv10 S19 S21 S36

Acute Entero-Colitis
Duodenitis B16 B17 B18 G24 Cv12 S25 S39 G41
Enteritis B22 B24 B25 Cv11 S25 Cv6 Li11 Li4 S37 S44

Colitis B22 B24 B25 B27 S25 Li10 S36 Li4 S37 S44
Proctitis B25 B27 B29 B30 B32 L5 Li4 S36 S44

Chronic Entero-Colitis
B22 B24 B25 Cv12 S25 Cv6 S28 S36

Appendicitis
Sp10 B54 Sp9 Sp8 Sp6 Liv2 T10 Li11 Li4 Appendix point S36.5

Intestinal Tuberculosis—only early stage
B20 B22 B24 B25 S25 Cv6 S36 Sp6

Intestinal Hernia?
Cv6 S25 S36 Sp6 Liv2
or B20 B22 B24 B25 S25 Cv4 S37 S36 Sp6

Constipation
Atonic B22 B24 B25 S25 Sp16 Cv3 T6 S36 Liv1
Habitual B25 B27 B33 S25 K16 S26 Cv9 T6 S36 B57 Sp3

Duodenal Ulcer
B11 B17 B18 B20 K21 S21 Cv12 P6 S36

Diarrhoea
B22 B25 S34 S25 Cv6 S36

Spastic Colitis
B24 B25 B31 S25 Cv6 S27 S28 S37

Proctitis
B31 B32 B29 Li10 Li4 S36 Sp6 Liv2

Haemorrhoids
Gv1 Gv3 B33 the two whites Sp6

Peritonitis (mediocre results)
Sp10 S36 Sp6 Liv2

Ascites (variable results)
B15 B22 B24 Cv9 Cv4 S28 Sp9 G38 Sp6 Liv2 G41
or B18 B23 B26 S25 Cv6 S27 Sp8 S36 S39 G39 K7 S44 Liv3

Cirrhosis
B16 B18 B20 B23 Liv14 Liv9 Sp9
or B17 B19 B22 B24 Liv13 Sp10 Sp6

Infectious Jaundice
Gv12 Gv9 B20 B43 B45 Li10 Si4 S36 S40 S44

Jaundice
B11 B17 B18 B20 B42 B43 Gv12 Gv9 Sp6

Biliary Colic
B18 B19 Si4 G34 G41 Liv2

Splenomegaly
B18 B20 B44 Cv12 Liv13 Cv6 S36

Acute Nephritis
B10 B12 B23 B25 B31 Liv13 T5 Li4 Sp9 Sp6

Chronic Nephritis
B22 B24 B25 B31 Cv6 S36 Sp9
or B23 B26 B32 S25 Cv4 Sp6

Pyelitis
B23 B25 B54 Sp10 S36 Sp6 K5

Cystitis
B25 B19 B31 B33 S36 Sp10 Sp9 Sp6

Haematuria
B23 B27 Cv6 Cv4 P7 L7 K7

Paralysis of Bladder
G33 B32 B33 Cv4 Cv3 Cv2

Spasm of Bladder
B25 B32 Cv6 Cv4 K10 G37 Liv8 Sp6 Liv3

Bladder Stone
B23 B28 Cv6 Cv4 Cv3 Sp9 Sp6

Nocturnal Enuresis
Gv20 B23 Gv4 Cv4

Stress Incontinence
Gv20 Gv4 B33 Cv4

Urethritis
Cv4 L7 Liv8 Sp6

Impotence
Gv20 B17 B21 B23 Gv4 Gv3 Cv4 Cv3

Nocturnal Emission
B15 B23 Gv3 Cv4 Cv1 Sp6

Orchitis
Li10 Li4 Liv8 Sp6 Liv4 Liv1

Prostatitis
Acute Cv6 Sp10 Sp9 Sp6 L9 K3
Chronic Gv2 Cv3 Gv20 K12 Sp6

Gonorrhoea
Acute B27 Cv6 Liv8 Sp6 Liv2 Li4
Chronic B27 B33 Cv3 Cv2 Sp6

DISEASES OF THE NERVOUS SYSTEM

Cerebral Anaemia
Gv20 G20 B20 Cv4 S36

Hypertensive Encephalopathy
G20 B10 Gv26 Li4 Li1 B60 B67
Mild paralysis of face, hand and leg Gv20 G20 T17 Li15 G34 S6 S7 S4

Cerebral Haemorrhage or Thrombosis
G20 B10 B11 G21 Li15 Li11 Li4 G30 G34 Sp6 B60

Chronic Headache

General points used in all varieties G20 B11 Li4 B62
Summit headache add Gv20 Gv21 Gv19 Si3
Frontal headache add Gv23 G14 S40 S44
Supraorbital headache add B2 G14 XH3
Unilateral headache add S8 XH3 G5 G4 G41

Cerebral Arterio-Sclerosis

Gv20 G21 Gv14 Li15 Li4 G38 B60 Liv2

Migraine

G20 S1 XH3 S7 S40 B60
Supplementary G15 G12 T22 G5 G6 B12 B14 T17 Cv13 Cv12 G41 L7 Liv2

Epilepsy with Fever

Cramps with fever, uraemia, plumbism, eclampsia, pneumonia in children, measles, acute fever, indigestion, intestinal parasites, teething.
G20 B10 Gv12 Cv13 (Cv10 and S25 not in pregnancy) Li11 Li1 S36 S45

Grand and Petit Mal, Violent Madness and Non-Violent Madness

G20 B13 B15 Cv15 Cv12 Cv6 H7 S40 Sp6
Don't exhaust oneself; no smoking; no drinking; restrict meat, especially beef, lamb, chicken; preferably vegetarian diet; reduce sex.

Writer's Cramp and similar conditions

G20 Li11 T5 T4 Li4 Si3

Carpo-Pedal Spasm

Hand Li11 L6 Li4 P7
Foot B60 S41 G41 S43

Chorea
G20 Gv14 Li11 T5 Li4 Si3
or B10 Gv12 Li10 G38 B60 S41

Athetosis
Hand Li11 L5 P7 P8 Si3 Li4
Foot S41 B60 K6 B63 K1

Parkinson's Disease
G20 Gv12 Gv4 Cv12 Cv4 L5 Si3
or B10 B11 Gv9 Cv13 Cv6 L6 B62

Travel Sickness
G20 B10 Cv12 Cv6 S36 S40 S44

Polyneuritis
Hand T5 P7 Li4 Si3 knuckles
Feet S41 B60 K6 toe knuckles

Occipital Neuralgia
G20 B11 G12 T5 Li4 S40 B60

Trigeminal Neuralgia
G20 T17 S7 Li10 Li4
Add for 1st division G14 B2
Add for 2nd   ,,   XH3 S2 S3
Add for 3rd   ,,   S5 S6

*Radial Nerve Neuralgia
B11 Si14 Li12 Li5 B10 Si13 T12 Li10 Li4

* Neuralgia, paralysis or spasm of a named nerve refers to:
1. Pain in the approximate distribution of this nerve.
2. Muscle weakness of the muscles innervated by this nerve.
3. Muscle spasm or cramps of the muscles innervated by the named nerve. The areas
   described are only very approximate.

Median Nerve Neuralgia
B10 Si13 P2 P4 P6

Ulnar Nerve Neuralgia
B10 Si13 H2 H6 H8

Anterior Thoracic Nerve Neuralgia
B10 Si13 S13 S15 L5 B11 Li15 S14 S16 S36

Long Thoracic Nerve Neuralgia
B11 Si14 L1 Sp19 Sp17 L5

Suprascapular Nerve Neuralgia
B11 Si14 Si12 T10 Si15 Si13 Si10 H3

Upper Subscapular Nerve Neuralgia
Si13 Si10 Si11 Li15

Circumflex Nerve Neuralgia
Li15 Si9 H1 T12

Intercostal Neuralgia
B11 B12 B13 B15 B18 K22 K25 L5 L9

Lumbago
B22 B25 B47 G26 G30 S31
or B23 B27 B46 G28 G29 Liv11

Sciatica (stationary pain)
B23 B25 Sp11 Sp9 Sp6 K4 Sp2

Sciatica (moving pain)
B32 G30 B50 B51 B54 G34 B55 Sp6 B60

Lateral Cutaneous Nerve of the Thigh Neuralgia
G30 G31 G32 G34

Obturator Nerve Neuralgia
Liv10 Sp11 Liv8 Sp6 Liv11 Liv9 K6 Sp9

Pudendal Nerve Neuralgia
B23 B25 B31 B32 Cv1 Sp6 Liv2

Joint Pain without Swelling
Knee XL2 B54 S33 G34 Sp6 B60
Wrist T4 Si5 Li5 Li4 T3 T5

Facial Palsy
S7 S6 S4 Cv24 Li4

Mandibular Nerve Paralysis
Gv20 G20 T17 T21 S6 S7 S4 Li4

Sublingual Nerve Paralysis
G20 B10 G21 Li17 Cv23 P7 H5

Strabismus
G20 B10 T17 XH3 B1 G5 Si6

Torticollis
G12 T16 Si16 G21 Si4 Si8

Radial Nerve Paralysis
G21 Li15 Li11 Li9 T4 L10 Li3
or Li16 T13 Li10 L6 Li5 L11 Li4

Median Nerve Paralysis
B10 Si15 G21 L3 P3 P4 P7 P8

Ulnar Nerve Paralysis
Si15 G21 Si13 T14 T10 Si8 Si7 H7 Si3

Long Thoracic Nerve Paralysis
B10 Si14 L1 Sp19 P1

Rhomboid Nerve Paralysis
B11 Si15 Si13 B13 B36 Li11
or Si14 G21 Si12 Si10 B12 T10

Upper Subscapular Nerve Paralysis
Si13 Si9 Li15 Li11 Si11 Si10 T14 T13

Circumflex Nerve Paralysis
B10 B11 Li15 T14 Li16 Li11

Paralysis of Diaphragm
B17 B18 G25 Liv13 S19 Cv6 S36 Sp6

Anterior Thoracic Nerve Paralysis
B10 B11 Si15 K27 K25 K23 S14 S16

Paralysis of Abdominal Muscles
Gv4 Gv3 B20 B22 B23 B25 Cv12 Cv6 S36 Sp6

Paralysis of Thigh
B23 B25 B31 B20 S33 Liv8 Sp4 Sp9

Obturator Nerve Paralysis
B23 B25 B29 G30 B50 B54 B57 Sp6
or B26 B32 B49 B51 B57 G34 G38 S41

Tibial Nerve Paralysis
B25 B31 B50 Sp11 Sp9 Sp6 K3
or B26 B32 Sp9 Liv8 B57 K6 Sp5

Peroneal Nerve Paralysis
B25 B32 G30 S36 G38 B60 B65
or B26 B31 B49 G34 B59 B62 B67

Facial Tic
G20 B10 T17 Li10 Li4

Sublingual Nerve Spasm
G20 B10 Gv16 Cv23 Li10 P7

Mandibular Nerve Spasm
G20 B10 T17 S7 S6 T5 S45

Spasm of Neck Muscles
G20 B10 G12 Li10 Si4

Spasm of Gastrocnemius
B57 B60

Hiccough
S10 Cv17 Cv14 Cv4

Spasm of Diaphragm
Cv14 Liv14 P6

Polyneuritis
Use local points as in sections on neuralgia and paralysis.
Add Gv14 Gv12 Gv9 B14 B16 Li11 T5 G34 B60

Beri-Beri
G31 S32 S35 XL2 S36 S37 S39 G39 G21 B15 B20 B23 B26 Cv9 Sp9 Sp6

Angio-Neurotic Oedema
Gv12 B17 B18 B25 Li15 Li11 Sp10 Sp6

Neurasthenia
G20 B11 B15 B22 Cv4 P6 S36
or B10 Gv12 B14 B23 Cv6 H5 Sp6

Violent Madness
Cv15 Cv12 Gv26 L11 Sp1 P7 B62 Gv16 S6 Cv24 P8 Gv23 H7 S36 S40

Non-Violent Madness—Singing, crying, happy, sad, senseless talk, cannot distinguish clean from dirty, lives in dream world, likes to sleep, behaves as drunk or crazy.
Cv15 G20 B13 B18 H7 Li4 Cv12 Cv6 S36 S40
or Cv13 B10 B15 B17 Si3 P4 H5 Cv4 S37 Sp6

Hysteria
B13 B15 B22 B32 Cv12 Cv4 Sp6
Treat every 2 or 3 days
If epileptic-like attack during treatment Cv17 Cv12 Cv6 P7

Acute and Chronic Rheumatoid Arthritis
Gv14 B11 Li15 Li11 T5 Li4
Plus local points 3 to 6 cm away from pain

Muscular Rheumatism
In loin B22 B24 B46 B31 B54
or B23 B25 B47 B32 S36
In neck G20 B10 Si15 Si14 T10 Si4
In scapular and interscapular area B36 B13 B39 B15 B40 B42
or B37 B12 B38 B14 B41 B18
In shoulders Li16 T15 Li15 Li14 T13 T14
Of pectoralis major and minor S13 S15 Sp20 G23 Li10 G34
or S14 S16 Sp19 Sp21 Li11 S36

Arthritis of Knee
S33 Liv8 Liv7 XL2 G34 Sp6 Sp9

Myositis
Gv14 Gv12 B20 Li11 T5 Li4 S36 Sp6

Gout
B23 B24 B19 Cv4 Sp6
Plus local points

Paget's Disease
Gv12 Gv9 Gv8 B13 B15 B20 B22 Li10 S36 Sp6

Vaginitis and Leucorrhoea
B32 Cv3 K12 Sp10 Sp6 Liv4 B31/4

Pruritis Vulvae
B25 B32 Gv1 Cv3 S30 Sp10 Sp6 B31/4

Acute and Chronic Endometritis
B23 B25 B32 B35 Liv8 Sp7 K4 B24 B27 B33 B30 Sp10 Sp6 Sp5

Acute and Chronic Metritis
B23 B31 Gv2 Cv3 Sp10 S37 Sp8 B24 B33 B35 Cv2 Sp9 S39 Sp6

Perimetritis
B31 B33 Cv6 S36 Sp6 Sp5 Sp3

Cancer of Cervix and Body of Womb (only secondary to radium etc.)
Cv4 Cv3 Cv2 B32 B33 B34 Gv2

Myoma
B32 (deep) Cv3 Liv5 Sp6 Liv2
or B33 (deep) Cv2 Liv6 K8 Liv3
If anaemic B17 B20 Cv4

Spasm of Uterus
B32 B33 S25 Cv6 S29 Cv2 Sp6

Abnormal Uterine Bleeding and Menorrhagia
Sp6 Sp1

Oophoritis
Acute S25 G26 Sp6
Chronic B24 B25 S25 K15 G26 S27 Sp6

Mastitis—particularly due to injury from breast feeding, not abscesses
S16 S18 G21 P3 S37 Liv3

Breast Pain—due to: too much milk, injury, anaemia, sex diseases, hysteria
B18 S14 S16 S18 Cv17 P1 H3

Nausea and Vomiting of Pregnancy
G20 B18 B25 B32 Cv17 S19 K15
or B10 B19 B27 B33 Cv16 S20 G26

Habitual Abortion
Gv4 B23 Gv3 S28 S36 Sp6

Dysmenorrhoea
Cv4 Cv3 S27 S28 Sp10 Sp6

Amenorrhoea
Gv4 B26 B32 Gv4 G26 Sp8 G33
or B23 B33 Gv3 K15 Sp6

DISEASES OF CHILDREN

Epileptic-Like Fits
Gv20 G20 Gv12 Li10 Li4 S36 Liv2

Pertussis
G20 Gv14 B12 Cv22 Cv13 L9 S36
alternate with B10 Gv12 B13 K27 Cv12 L8 S40

Meningitis
G20 Gv14 Gv7 B23 S25 S36
alternate with B10 Gv12 Gv4 B22 Cv6 G34

ENDOCRINE DISEASES

Goitre and Myxoedema
G20 Gv14 B11 Cv22 S10 Gv4 T3
or B10 Gv12 B12 Cv23 S9 Gv3 G26

Addison's Disease
B22 B23 both 2 Chinese inches deep Gv6 Gv5 S25 Sp14

Diabetes—mild
B13 B18 B20 B23 Cv23 Cv12 Cv4 L9 H7 Sp6 K2

Diabetes Insipidus
B22 B24 B23 Cv4

DISEASES OF THE EYES

Conjunctivitis
G20 B2 B1 XH3 Li4 G37

Night Blindness
B18 B19 G20 B1 Li4 S36
or B42 B43 G12 B2 Li10 G37

Blepharitis
B2 B1 S2 G1 Mid dorsal surface of interphalangeal joint of thumb, mid dorsal surface of proximal interphalangeal joint of little finger, prick eyelids till blood flows.

Dacryocystitis
B2 B1 S2 G14 B18 B22 G8

Trachoma
G14 B2 G1 G20 B18 Si19 G37 G42

EAR, NOSE AND THROAT DISEASES

Otitis Media
G20 T17 T21 Li11 Li4
Better result when surgery and acupuncture combined

Sinusitis
G20 Si15 Gv23 Li20 Li10 Li4 B17

Hay Fever, Allergic Rhinorrhoea, Influenza
G20 B10 Gv23 Li20 Li4
In chronic cases add Gv20 B7 Gv23 B12

Epistaxis
G20 Si15 Gv23 Li4 S36 Liv3

INFECTIONS

Dysentery (only assists medical treatment)
B25 B29 Li4 S37 Gv14 Gv12

Typhoid (before fluid loss only)
XA1 B54 L5 Cv13 Cv12 Cv6 S25 S36 B57

Bubonic Plague (helped in outbreak in Fookin province in Sino-Japanese war 1940)
Pierce skin with three-cornered needle over axillary and groin glands, till blood flows. L5 B54 Li11 Li4 T5 S36 S44 XA1 all till blood flows.

Meningitis (Subsidiary treatment. Reduces intracranial pressure and muscle spasm).
Gv8 Gv8.5 Gv9 G20 B11 to 19 Cv21 Cv17 Cv13 Cv12 Cv10 Li11 Li4 Li1 L11 P9 H9 Si1 T1 K1 B67 Liv1 G44 S45 Sp1 B54 B57 B60 Liv2 S44 all just pricked without leaving needle in place

Malaria (subsidiary treatment)
Gv14 P5 Si3 K7
In chronic cases add B20 B23 Gv4 Cv4

Cold
G20 B13 Gv12 T5
With nasal symptoms add Gv23 Li4
With laryngeal symptoms add T2 L10
With bronchitis add L9 L5
For those who get colds easily B12 B13 S36 daily for one month

Influenza (symptomatic treatment)
Headache G20 G15 B2 S8
Muscular aches Li11 T5 G34 B60
Epistaxis Li4
Nose blocked Gv23
Dry cough L9
Pain in throat L10
Vomits Cv12 S36
Constipation S25
Delirious P5 S44
Body stiff Gv14 Gv12 Gv9
To reduce fever Gv14 Gv12 Li11 Li4 S36 S44

Periosteal Acupuncture

Over the past nine years I have evolved an acupuncture technique which I have christened periosteal acupuncture. It is particularly efficacious in diseases of the joints.

The technique is simple, though in some instances it requires a good knowledge of anatomy. An acupuncture or hypodermic needle is used. The needle at the appropriate place, pierces the soft tissue surrounding the joint and then stimulates the periosteum. The periosteum is 'pecked', much as a woodpecker pecks a tree, till the required degree of stimulation has been achieved.

If mild stimulation is required I use a 30 or 28-gauge stainless steel acupuncture needle and 'peck' only lightly for a short time. When stronger stimulation is appropriate a 25, 23, 21, or even 19-gauge disposable hypodermic needle may be used. The hypodermic needles being hollow are more rigid than acupuncture needles so that the 'pecking' may be done with considerable force, sometimes bending the tip of the needle. If one expects the procedure to be unduly painful (which is rare except with a calcaneal spur or occasionally with the greater trochanter or lateral epicondyle of the humerus) a local anaesthetic may be used. I use 2% xylocaine without adrenaline, injected at the surface of the periosteum. 1 cc or less is sufficient and after a delay of about a minute the more violent type of 'pecking' may commence.

In a patient who has say cervical osteoarthritis with resultant brachial neuralgia, a needle stimulating the transverse process of a lower cervical vertebra, will in the appropriate case alleviate the symptoms. If the needle does not stimulate the periosteum, but instead stimulates the overlying skin or muscles, or hits one of the nerves of the brachial plexus (producing a shooting pain down the arm), the result is in most instances not so good. I have repeatedly stimulated the skin, muscle, or a major nerve trunk over a joint and found it as a rule not as effective as when the periosteum is stimulated in the correct place.

It is well known that there are more nerve fibres and endings in the skin and periosteum than in most other tissues and hence a needle piercing the skin or periosteum hurts more than when passing through the intervening subcutaneous tissue or muscles. I assume there is a local nerve network in the periosteum surrounding the joints and innervating their structures. And I also assume that the nerves in the muscles and skin only communicate with the periosteal nerve network somewhat sparsely. This theory could explain why stimulating the periosteum of joints has a greater effect than pricking the skin. On the other hand, if a disease does not involve a joint, stimulating the skin or periosteum have an equal effect for an equal strength of stimulation.

I would be interested to hear of any histological or physiological research that has been done concerning the above theory.

Whether or not the conditions mentioned below respond, depends mainly on the degree and reversibility of the pathological changes. Although the intra-articular bone rarely regenerates, the positions of the bones relative to one another may be altered by varying the pull of the attached muscles, and hence alleviate temporarily or even permanently the patient's symptoms.

TRANSVERSE PROCESS OF LOWER CERVICAL VERTEBRAE (near Si16)

There are many patients who have pain at the back of the neck, in the occipital area, over the shoulders and down the arms to the fingers. There may be limitation of movement of the neck with crepitus.

A fairly high proportion of these patients may be helped, often even considerably, provided the main symptom is pain. When there are more objective signs, such as paraesthesia, anaesthesia, diminished reflexes, loss of muscular strength and muscle wasting, the chances of success are considerably diminished, though not hopeless—one's clinical judgement being of paramount importance. I imagine the pain is more easily alleviated than the more objective signs, as pain is produced by a milder degree of nerve root compression and hence quite often the pathology is presumably less severe. I would be interested to hear the comments of others on this theory.

The stiffness of the neck may also be alleviated, according to its pathology. Restriction of sideways movement and rotation is easier to alleviate than flexion and extension.

A 30-gauge acupuncture needle is the best. Do not use a hypodermic needle as these are sharpened in such a way as to produce a cutting edge, which cuts its way through the tissues and blood vessels and may thus produce a haematoma. An acupuncture needle is pushed through the tissue like a wedge and hence only rarely causes bleeding.

The transverse processes at the side of the neck are palpated by pressing the overlying muscles firmly against the bone. The greatest tenderness is usually at the level of the 5th or 6th cervical vertebra on the affected side.

The transverse process of maximal tenderness is selected. The needle pierces the overlying skin and muscles going in horizontally and at right angles to the neck. *For this technique, more than any other, the relevant anatomy must first be studied.**

It is often surprisingly difficult to hit the transverse process, the needle passing anteriorly or posteriorly. An accurate assessment should be made of the depth of the tip of the transverse process in each patient, and if this

* The books I refer to continuously are: J. C. Boileau Grant, 'An Atlas of Anatomy', Williams & Williams, Baltimore. Johannes Sobotta, 'Atlas of Descriptive Human Anatomy', Hafner Publishing Co., New York. (In German: Urban & Schwarzenberg, Munich-Berlin). Eduard Pernkopf, 'Atlas of Topographical and Applied Human Anatomy', W. B. Saunders Co., Philadelphia. (In German: Urban & Schwarzenberg, Munich-Berlin). 'Gray's Anatomy', Longmans, London.

depth is exceeded the needle partially or totally withdrawn and reinserted to find the tip of the transverse process. The vertebra should not be 'pecked' too vigorously.

All the lower cervical vertebrae may be stimulated in the above manner. It is perhaps safer to avoid stimulating the transverse processes of the upper cervical vertebrae considering the more intricate anatomy.

GREATER TROCHANTER (G30)

Mild osteoarthritis of the hip may be alleviated for a few years by needling the greater trochanter. Total replacement of the hip joint is of course the only final answer, but often the degree of pain or limitation of movement does not warrant such a major operation. These mild cases may not too infrequently be helped, but only to a moderate degree. Often the pathology advances and something more drastic has to be done later. There are some patients with pain in the region of the hip joint with a negative X-ray. These patients can be cured, though some of them develop osteoarthritis a few years later.

Although a fine acupuncture needle may be used in the mildest cases or in hypersensitive patients, a thicker hypodermic needle is more often appropriate. Mostly I use a 21-gauge $1\frac{1}{2}''$ needle. In fat patients a 19-gauge $2''$ needle is needed. The greater trochanter apparently moves nearer the surface, thus facilitating needling, with the patient supine. On rare occasions a local anaesthetic is advised.

K5 and G40 on the opposite side may also be used. Also G30 and G26. Liv9 ipsilaterally helps groin pain on abduction.

CORACOID PROCESS (near L1)

The so-called frozen shoulder may be helped or cured by stimulating the coracoid process. If the patient can raise his arm only a few degrees, this method will not help. It is useful though in moderate and mild cases.

The tip of the coracoid process is 'pecked' with either an acupuncture needle or a 25 or 23-gauge disposable hypodermic. The needle is held horizontally and pierces the skin overlying the tip of the coracoid process.

If the above does not have an immediate effect, needling the transverse process of a tender cervical vertebra may help, for there often seems to be an association. The biceps tendon in the bicipital groove may be palpated for a tender area and needled. Otherwise one may use Li15 Si9 Si10 L5 P3.

It is also important to exercise the shoulder by asking the patient to do those movements he cannot do or finds painful. Swinging the arm in an arc that does not cause pain is in my experience useless. The painful and restricted movements should be forced to such an extent that the patient has tears in his eyes and the movements should be repeated several times a day. The exercise should not be so severe as to cause aching in the shoulder for more than a few minutes after the cessation of the exercise.

LATERAL EPICONDYLE OF HUMERUS (near Li12)

A reasonable, but not too high, proportion of patients with a tennis elbow may be helped or cured by needling the lateral epicondyle of the humerus.

The epicondyle is easiest felt with the elbow at a right angle. A 25-gauge needle is the best size.

If the above procedure does not help, needling Gv14 very strongly may help. Sometimes the neck is also implicated, in which case the appropriate tender transverse process of a cervical vertebra should be stimulated. The following may also be tried: Li4 Li14 Li15 all on the affected side.

A cortisone injection is sometimes more effective. I suspect this is due to its strong irritant properties, for the patient often has severe pain for the following two days, whilst with acupuncture the pain wears off in seconds or minutes. It could be said that cortisone injected at the correct place is no more than powerful acupuncture. It has though the disadvantage that it may cause a small localised area of necrosis, which normal acupuncture does not.

An injection of a local anaesthetic at the appropriate place is of greater benefit whilst the anaesthetic lasts, but afterwards has no greater effect than a dry needle.

If the pain is over the medial epicondyle or the olecranon process, these should instead be needled. As additional stimulation (instead of using large intestine points), one should use in the former instance heart and small intestine and in the latter instance triple warmer acupuncture points.

If the tennis elbow is due to an entrapment lesion, an operation is necessary.

CALCANEAL SPUR

The pain that may be caused by a calcaneal spur or plantar fasciitis may be cured in a high proportion of patients.

The tender area is localised with strong digital pressure on the heel. A 23 or more often 21-gauge needle is used and 1 cc of 2% xylocain is injected down to the bone. The bone is then 'pecked' with considerable strength in the case of a spur and more gently with plantar fasciites. Not infrequently the patient may have some pain for three days afterwards due to the strength of stimulation that is required for this procedure to be effective, and also presumably due to the heel being dependent and walked on. K3 K4 B62 B61 occasionally help.

SACRO-ILIAC JOINT (B26)

A large proportion of patients with low backache or sciatica may be helped by needling the sacro-iliac joint.

Mostly I ask the patient to sit in a chair and lean forwards. A 21-gauge needle is inserted in or near the dimple which overlies the joint. The needle is pushed into the joint between the sacrum and the ileum, which often necessitates touching the bone on either side of the joint till one finds the space between the bones.

This technique works (as with the transverse process of the cervical vertebrae) if the main symptom is pain in the lumbar or sacral area, or is of sciatic distribution. The chances of success are considerably diminished when there is anaesthesia, paraesthesia, muscle weakness or wasting, reduced reflexes, or there are trophic changes.

I assume acupuncture is of benefit in these conditions as it alters the tone of the lumbar muscles, thus altering the alignment of the vertebrae and hence relieves pressure on the nerve roots. I would be interested to hear of readers' comments on this.

In some instances other acupuncture points (acupuncture points do not exist—but one has to describe something) are more effective. My favourite ones at the moment are Liv3 and B62, though there is a choice of about twenty acupuncture points, depending on the distribution of pain or other symptoms and also on the findings of pulse diagnosis.

If a patient has advanced pelvic malignant disease with pain over the sacrum, but anaesthesia of the legs due to involvement of the lumbo-sacral plexus by the tumour, normal acupuncture does not work. Normally with sacral pain one might stimulate B62, but clearly this does not work when the nerve has been interrupted. In this instance an acupuncture point at the opposite end of the body such as B2 works very well.

BELOW MEDIAL CONYLE OF TIBIA (Sp9)

The majority of women have a small, tender oedematous area below the medial condyle of the tibia, a position which could be called Sp9. It is at the insertion of the medial ligament of the knee. Sometimes the tender area is 2 cm in diameter, sometimes there are one or several small areas.

The periosteum at this point may be stimulated gently or strongly according to the case.

This method is surprisingly effective in many painful conditions of the knee. Whether the pain be medial, lateral, anterior or posterior, it is the point of first choice.

Alternative points are G33 B54 peripatella points.

POSTERIOR SPINES OF LOWER LUMBAR VERTEBRAE

Skyrme Rees of Sydney considers that the pain of ordinary low backache and sciatica originates from the lumbar posterior intervertebral joints, the hypophyseal joints—this theory does not include genuine herniated intervertebral discs. The nerve supply to the posterior intervertebral joints arises from the posterior primary division of the segmental nerves, being the first extradural branch. Skyrme Rees divided the above nerves, in the appropriate segments, percutaneously, using a fine scalpel,* a method called rhizolysis.

Norman Shealy of Wisconsin, a neurosurgeon, from whom I first heard of this technique, modified Skyrme Rees' method. Under X-ray control, he inserted, percutaneously, a diathermy probe directly onto the posterior intervertebral joint.

Benjamin Cox of California, likewise a neurosurgeon, modified Norman Shealy's method, which likewise had been a modification of Skyrme Rees'. He inserted, percutaneously, under X-ray control, a dry needle and merely 'pecked' the posterior intervertebral joints.

After the above two doctors told me their methods, I tried to modify them in such a way as to be more easily applicable to the practice of a general practitioner using acupuncture:

Using a 28-gauge 2″ acupuncture needle, I needled, without X-ray control, the posterior intervertebral joint. The result was good, but difficult

---

* *The Treatment of Pain as the Major Disability* by W. Skyrme Rees 1975. Visual Abstracts (Australia) Pty., Sydney.

to perform, except in the thinnest of patients. I was also not too sure that the needle was always in the correct position.

Later I stimulated instead the lamina of the lower lumbar vertebrae: a simpler technique with equally good results.

Most recently I have merely stimulated the posterior spinous process. I ask the patient to sit on a chair, leaning forward, to produce a slight kyphosis in the lumbar area. The posterior spine is palpated and a 28-gauge 2″ acupuncture needle is inserted about one inch laterally. The needle is angled in such a way that the lateral side of the spine is stimulated, rather nearer the lamina than the tip of the spinous process. As the spinal cord terminates at L2, I only use the above technique for the lower three lumbar vertebrae. Above this level I use a modification—see below.

A comparison of the results obtained by Skyrme Rees, with the modifications of Norman Shealy, Benjamin Cox and myself is difficult, as all four methods depend to a considerable extent on the skill of the individual doctor. The experience of my own practice and the heresay of colleagues suggests the results are similar, though I know several doctors prefer one method to another.

G. S. Hackett has for many years used a related technique in which a sclerosing solution is injected into, and around, various ligaments in the lumbar and sacral area, a method called prolotherapy. Some doctors who used these sclerosing solutions for several years, have since tried my periosteal needling techniques, and have found that both methods produce similar results.

POSTERIOR SPINES OF THORACIC VERTEBRAE AND UPPER LUMBAR VERTEBRAE

The posterior spines of the above vertebrae may be stimulated by a slight modification of the technique described for the lower lumbar vertebrae. Due to the proximity of the spinal cord, I needle the lateral side of the spinous process somewhat nearer the tip of the spinous process (whilst for the lower lumbar vertebrae it was somewhat nearer the lamina). In the upper lumbar and lower thoracic region I still use a 28-gauge 2″ needle. In the upper thoracic area, where the spinous processes are nearer the surface I use a 30-gauge 1″ needle, piercing the skin only $\frac{1}{2}$″ lateral to the midline.

The needle may also be inserted in the midline so that the tip of the spinous process is stimulated. At the moment I am inclined to think that the results of this method are not quite as good as when the lateral side of the spinous process is needled.

The upper lumbar and thoracic vertebrae may be stimulated in painful conditions, which one thinks are of vertebral origin and of a partially reversible nature.

Stimulating the transverse processes of the cervical vertebrae may often be used for treating pain in the head, neck and even interscapular area down to a level of T6 or 7. Treatment of the sacro-iliac joint, the ischial tuberosity or the lumbar vertebrae often helps in the ordinary types of lumbago or sciatica. Neither of the above methods though, help pain in the lower half of the thoracic area, which is best treated by stimulating the tender vertebrae. Interscapular pain, as mentioned above, is often referred from the cervical area, and should then of course be treated via the cervical vertebrae. Sometimes interscapular pain is of upper thoracic origin, in which case the appropriate thoracic vertebrae should be treated.

ISCHIAL TUBEROSITY

The patient is asked to sit on a chair and lean as far foward as possible. A second chair may be placed in front of him so that the patient may lean his arms or head on it. The ischial tuberosity is palpated and 'pecked' with a 28-gauge 2″ needle.

This method helps selected patients with low backache and suprisingly enough patients with pain in the knee. On a few ocassions it helps coccydynia, though at the time of writing I still do not have a satisfactory answer for most cases.

TEMPERO-MANDIBULAR JOINT

The patient is asked to open and close his mouth several times, so that the head of the mandible may be palpated, and most particularly the joint space above it identified. A 30-gauge 1″ needle is inserted into the joint space.

This technique may be used in patients with mild pain in the tempero-mandibular joint. Sometimes orthodontic treatment is more satisfactory.

Catarrh of the eustachian tube occasionally responds.

There are some patients who have pain below the eye, along or just below the inferior orbital margin. This may respond to needling the tempero-mandibular joint, suggesting it is pain referred from this joint. On a few occasions even pain anywhere in the cheek, or mandible may respond, possibly even supraorbital pain.

FIRST METACARPO-PHALANGEAL JOINT

Osteoarthritis may develop in the joint, with a tender nodule over its lateral aspect. Sometimes local needling helps.

LIVER AND ABDOMINAL SYMPTOMS

One of the commonest symptoms I treat are patients who are 'livery'. I use the word in its French rather than in the Anglo-Saxon sense, which is described in detail in my book *Meridians of Acupuncture*.

This may not infrequently be helped by needling the periosteum or perichondrium of the lower ribs. I usually stimulate in the mid-nipple line between the inferior margin of the breast and the lower costal margin. The nearest, non-existent acupuncture point, would be liver 14.

If the patient's symptoms involve the lower abdomen, the anterior superior iliac spine may be pecked. Sometimes the rib point mentioned above as well as the anterior superior iliac spine are needled.

STERNUM, MANUBRIUM, ANTERIOR RIBS

The above may be stimulated in mild conditions of the chest involving bronchospasm.

Usually I needle the sternum or manubrium anywhere in the midline. Sometimes I needle in the region of the costo-chondral junction of the 2nd and 3rd ribs.

The needling of ribs may easily be performed in thin patients whose ribs can be palpated. Unless one is completely sure that one has been able to isolate a rib between two fingers, the procedure should not be performed.